Take Care of Yourself

A Health Care Workbook for Beginning ESL Students

Marianne Brems
Theresa Devonshire R. N.
Janet R. Jones

PRENTICE HALL REGENTS
Englewood Cliffs, New Jersey 07632

Brems, Marianne.
Take care of yourself: a health care workbook for beginning ESL
students / /by Marianne Brems, Theresa Devonshire, Janet Jones.
        p.   cm.
    Includes bibliographical references.
    ISBN 0-13-882317-0
    1. Health.   2. Medical care—United States.   3. English language—
-Textbooks for foreign speakers.   I. Devonshire, Theresa.
II> Jones, Janet (Janet R.)   III> Title.
RA776.5.B74 1994
362.1dc20   93-7377
                                                                  CIP

Acquisitions editor: *Nancy Leonhardt*
Managing editor: *Sylvia Moore*
Editorial/production supervision,
   and interior design: *Christine McLaughlin Mann*
Copyeditor: Virginia Rubens
Cover design: Yes Graphics
Interior Illustrations: *Gayle Levée*
Production Coordinator: *Ray Keating*

© 1994 by PRENTICE HALL REGENTS
Prentice Hall, Inc.
A Paramount Communications Company
Englewood Cliffs, New Jersey 07632

Printed in the United States of America

10   9   8   7   6   5   4   3   2   1

ISBN   0-13-882317-0

Prentice-Hall International (UK) Limited, London
Prentice-Hall of Australia Pty. Limited, Sydney
Prentice-Hall Canada Inc., Toronto
Prentice-Hall Hispanoamericana, S.A., Mexico
Prentice-Hall of India Private Limited, New Delhi
Prentice-Hall of Japan, Inc., Tokyo
Simon & Schuster Asia Pte. Ltd., Singapore
Editora Prentice-Hall do Brasil, Ltda., *Rio de Janeiro*

Contents

Introduction

This book for adolescent and adult language students consists of 25 short health-care episodes lovingly created to represent real-life situations along with the real attitudes of real people. In this case the real people are members of the Santos family—a family, like so many in the United States, in which both husband and wife work, but are also parents.

In further keeping with reality, we have attempted to represent the modern roles of men and women in the United States—roles that may differ in some cases from those of men and women in other countries. For example, the reader sees that in our country men sometimes cook and women sometimes are doctors.

We have been particularly conscious of the interest level of the adolescent and adult language student, and we hope that our readers will enjoy seeing the characters unfold as we have.

We have also been conscious of the four major areas of health care, which include personal health care at home or away from the health care facility, community health care services, health care for children and adolescents, and women's health care.

In regard to the structure of the book, the sentences are not long or complicated, and although the lessons are not necessarily presented in order of difficulty, some of the earlier lessons are briefer and simpler. Simplicity, however, has been a main concern throughout, but not at the expense of authenticity.

In the interest of authenticity, the episodes are only very loosely grammar based. At all times, a higher priority has been placed on the use of language that is realistic and appropriate to the situation. A word list of health terms along with other common words used in the stories provides a basis for reading comprehension as well as for vocabulary building.

Each lesson includes information beyond that contained in the story, sometimes in the form of a "Cultural Note" that pays particular attention to the attitudes Americans have and the ways in which American health care representatives deal with specific health issues. All lessons present the most up-to-date information available.

The book is intended for use in the classroom, where students can interact with the teacher and with classmates, or outside of the classroom, where students can individually make use of the answer keys in the *Teacher's Manual* to check their work. Similarly the "What about you?" sections can likewise be used for class or small-group discussion or for individual introspection.

The overall objectives of the book are

- ○ To help the student develop the basic competencies necessary for proper health care
- ○ To help the student better understand American health care and health care attitudes
- ○ To help the student develop interest in reading
- ○ To help the student increase reading comprehension
- ○ To help the student build vocabulary useful in everyday life
- ○ To lay the ground work for critical thinking.

 # Acknowledgments

For consultation and provision of literature on many of the aspects of health care covered in this book, we wish to thank Abbey Goll-Keane of the San Mateo City Elementary School District, and the San Mateo County Department of Health Services, particularly Marilyn Jordan.

From Marianne Brems
To Holly Fulghum-Nutters who has been an inspiration and a special friend to me in my personal growth as an ESL teacher.

From Theresa Devonshire
To Mr. Spock, Captain Kirk, and the crew of the Starship Enterprise who boldly went where no man has gone before, and took me with them.

From Janet Jones
To my husband, Kip, with many thanks for not changing the word processing program on me (again) until my work on the book was finished.

Unit 1

Personal And Home Health Care

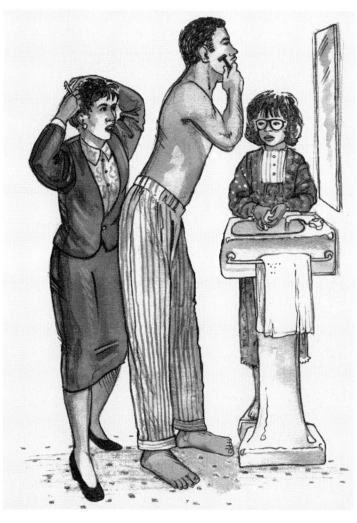

Daily Personal Hygiene

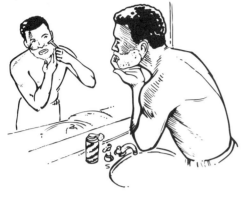

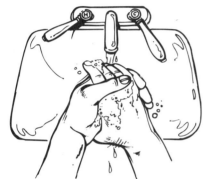

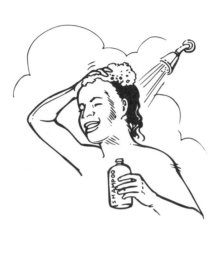

WORD LIST

Nouns **Things**

hygiene
shower
shampoo
soap
washcloth
mirror
deodorant
razor
shaving cream
nail clipper
comb

Descriptions

daily
personal

It's morning. Tomas is taking a shower before he goes to work. He's washing his hair with shampoo.

He's rubbing lots of soap on his washcloth. He's rubbing his whole body with the washcloth. He's washing his arms, legs, back, face, and ears. He's careful not to fall when he washes his feet.

He's rinsing off all the soap. He's closing his eyes tight. Soap in your eyes hurts!

He's standing in front of the bathroom mirror. He's putting on deodorant. He's shaving with a razor and shaving cream.

He's cutting his fingernails and toenails with a nail clipper.

He's combing his hair with a comb. Tomas's nine-year-old daughter, Cathy, is banging on the bathroom door and saying, "Daddy, hurry up! It's my turn in the bathroom."

Comprehension Check

Circle the correct answer.

1. Which part of the day is it?

   a. morning　　b. afternoon　　c. evening

2. Tomas is washing his hair with _____.

   a. a washcloth　　b. soap　　**c.** shampoo

3. Tomas is washing his body with _____.

   a. soap　　b. a razor　　c. shampoo

4. What is Tomas shaving with?

   a. a razor　　b. a nail clipper　　c. a comb

5. Who's banging on the door?

   a. Tomas　　b. Tomas's wife　　**c.** Tomas's daughter

Cultural Note

Many Americans shower every morning and wash their clothes after wearing them just one time. But that's not all. They wash their hands many times every day, too.

It's a good idea to wash your hands after touching pets, after touching someone who is sick, and after using the bathroom. Always wash your hands before cooking or eating.

Vocabulary Builder

Write the correct word from the list below under each picture.

deodorant	comb	razor	mirror
washcloth	shampoo	shower	shaving cream
nail clipper	soap		

_____razor_____

_____soap_____

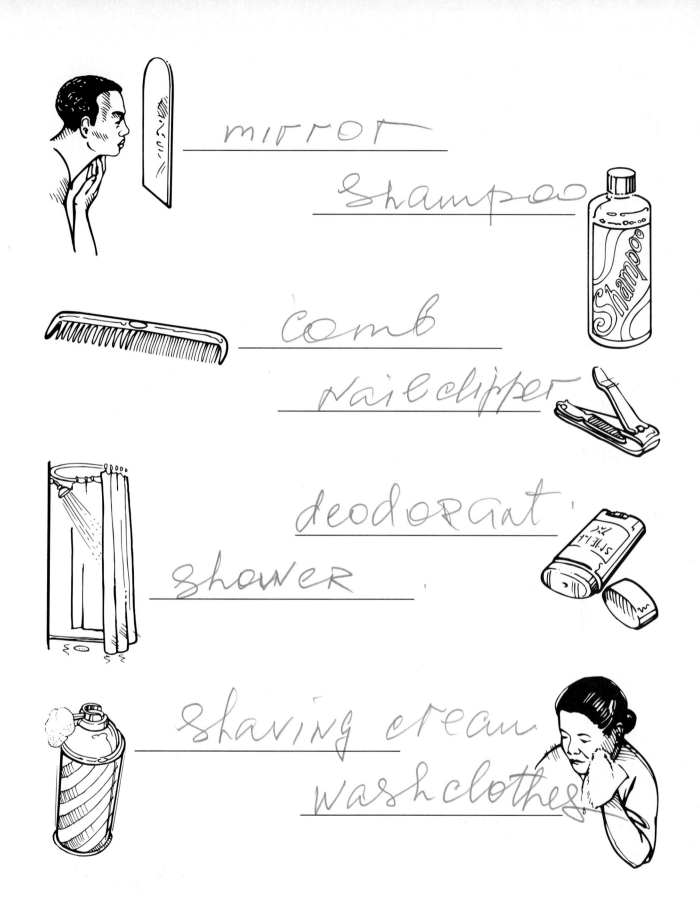

mirror

shampoo

comb

nail clipper

deodorant

shower

shaving cream

washclothes

Fill in the Blank

Write the correct words from the list below in the blanks.

mirror   soap   washcloth   nail clipper
razor   comb   shampoo   shaving cream

What is he/she using?

1. Kai is washing his hair. He is using _____ *shampoo* .
2. Naomi is cutting her fingernails. She is using a
   Nail clipper .
3. Lee is combing his hair. He is using a _____ *comb* _____ and a
   _____ *brush* .
4. Sarita is taking a shower. She is using _____ *soap* _____ and a
   washcloth
5. Thien is shaving. He is using a _____ *razor* _____ and
   shaving cream .

Activity

With another student, list which of the following items you need in the shower and which items you need outside the shower. Some items may go in both lists. Write the words below in the correct list. Compare your lists with other students' lists.

shampoo   mirror   shaving cream
soap   deodorant   nail clipper
washcloth   razor   comb

razor

In the shower

shampoo
soap
washcloth

Outside the shower

mirror
deodorant
RAZOR
shaving cream
nail clipper
comb .

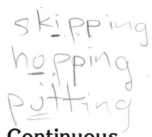 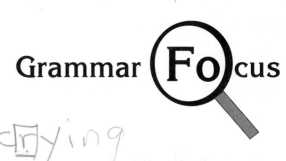

a e i o u.

skipping
hopping
putting

Grammar (Fo)cus

drying

Present Continuous

The present continuous is the tense used to describe an action that is going on right now. Form the present continuous by using the present-tense form of the verb "to be" and adding "ing" to the base form of the main verb.

For example: Ramon <u>is</u> wash<u>ing</u> his hands.

Fill in the blanks with the correct form of the verb to make sentences using the present continuous.

For example: He (cut) _____ _____ his fingernails.
He <u>is</u> <u>cutting</u> his fingernails.

1. Pham (take) _is taking_ a shower.
2. Ana (wash) _is washing_ her hands.
3. They (go) _are going_ to the movies with their friends.
4. Rogelio and Ida (have) _are having_ a party at their house.
5. She (put) _is putting_ her car in the garage.

What about you?

- ○ When do you wash your hands?
- ○ Do you always wash your hands even when you're in a hurry?
- ○ Are washing customs different in your country?

Reading comprehension grade 5
Vocabulary - 6.
9,10,11 - average
0 1 2 3 4 5 6 7 8 9 10 11 19

Let's Play Charades
(practice in asking questions)

The following activities will be written out on separate pieces of paper. The class will be divided into two teams. One person from each team will take turns acting out the personal hygiene activity written on the piece of paper which the teacher will hand out. In order to win a point, a member of that person's team must identify the activity *and* phrase the question correctly. Example: "Are you brushing your teeth?"

taking a bubble bath	putting on shaving cream
getting soap in your eyes	putting on deodorant
washing your hands	waking up
shaving	rubbing soap on a wash
clipping your nails	cloth
putting on makeup	banging on the door
taking a cold shower	taking a hot shower
combing your hair	standing in front of a mirror
washing your hair	washing behind your ears
doing the laundry (washing clothes)	

Commercials
(personal hygiene products)

Write the letter of the product in the blank before each problem.

_d_ dirty hair   a. soap

_a_ dirty skin   b. razor, shaving cream

_e_ bad breath   c. laundry detergent

_b_ heavy beard   d. shampoo

_c_ dirty clothes   e. toothpaste

In groups of 2, 3, or 4 people, prepare a 15-second commercial about one of the following products:

Nockumded Shampoo	Mr. Macho Shaving Cream
Barra Soap	Tuba Toothpaste
Sharpo Razors	Sudso Laundry Detergent

It is best if you make up your own words, but if that is too difficult, here are some ideas to help you. Your commercial could sound something like this:

Are you having a problem with ___*hair*___? Try our new, improved ___*shampoo*___ and then you will have no more problem. With our new, improved ___*shampoo*___ you will be able to ___*look good*___ and everyone in your family will be happy. Remember now, try ___*Wella Shampoo*___. Do it today!

Before or After?
(pair activity)

Find out if your partner knows which activities come before and which come after. Be prepared to report your findings to the class. Partner A asks Partner B questions. Partner B responds.

> **Example:**
> Partner A: Do you put on your shoes **before** your socks or **after**?
> Partner B: (a.) I put on my socks before I put on my shoes.
>   b. I put on my shoes after I put on my socks.

PARTNER A's QUESTIONS:

1. Do you brush your teeth before you go to bed or after?
2. Do you dry yourself off before you take a shower or after?
3. Do you get dressed before you take a shower or after?
4. Do you rub your skin with a washcloth before you put soap on it or after?
5. Do you put on deodorant before you wash yourself or after?
6. Do you wash your hands before you eat or after?
7. Do you wash your hands before you use the bathroom or after?

PARTNER B's RESPONSES:

1. a. I brush my teeth before I go to bed.
   b. I brush my teeth after I go to bed.
2. a. I dry myself off before I take a shower.
   b. I dry myself off after I take a shower.
3. a. I get dressed before I take a shower.
   b. I get dressed after I take a shower.
4. a. I rub my skin with a washcloth before I put soap on it.
   b. I rub my skin with a washcloth after I put soap on it.
5. a. I put on deodorant before I wash myself.
   b. I put on deodorant after I wash myself.
6. a. I wash my hands before I eat.
   b. I wash my hands after I eat.
7. a. I wash my hands before I use the bathroom.
   b. I wash my hands after I use the bathroom.

Oral Care

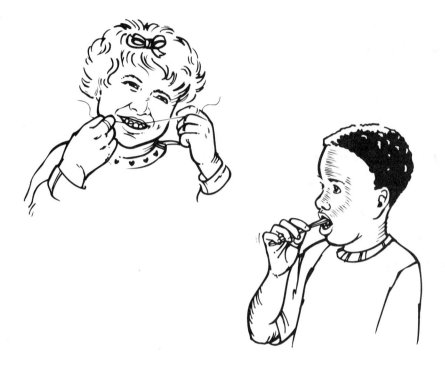

WORD LIST

Things

toothbrush
toothpaste
tongue
dental floss
plaque
gum disease
tooth decay
dental examination
dental insurance
gums
X-ray
mouthwash

Descriptions

oral

It's evening. Theresa is getting ready for bed. She's brushing her teeth with a toothbrush and toothpaste. She's brushing her tongue, too.

She's using dental floss to remove plaque from between her teeth. You can't see plaque, but it causes gum disease and tooth decay. Your teeth don't feel smooth and clean when they have plaque on them. To remove plaque, Theresa brushes her teeth every morning and every evening.

Every six months she goes to the dentist for an examination. She has dental insurance where she works. The dentist cleans her teeth and checks for tooth decay and gum disease. Sometimes he takes a special picture of Theresa's teeth called an X-ray. With an X-ray he can see inside her teeth and gums. He can find little problems with Theresa's teeth before they are big, expensive problems. He takes good care of Theresa's teeth. She never wakes up with a toothache. Good night, Theresa. Sleep well.

Comprehension Check

Circle the correct answer.

1. Which time of the day is it?

    a. morning   b. afternoon   (c.) evening

2. Theresa is brushing her teeth with a toothbrush
   and __toothpaste__ ?

    a. plaque   (b.) toothpaste   c. dental floss

3. To remove plaque between her teeth Theresa
   uses _____.

    a. toothpaste   (b.) dental floss   c. toothbrush

4. Theresa brushes her teeth _____.

    a. once a day   (b.) twice a day   c. every six months

5. Theresa has a dental examination every _____

    (a.) six months   b. month   c. year

6. A picture of your teeth is called a/an _____

    a. tooth decay   b. dental examination   (c.) X-ray

Cultural Note

Americans are often afraid their mouths smell bad to people they talk to. Many Americans use mouthwash in the morning and before going out with other people. Sometimes they carry little breath mints with them to eat when they're out. Americans don't like any bad smells.

Vocabulary Builder

Circle the correct word and write the word in the blank.

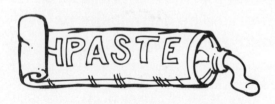

toothpaste   tooth decay
toothbrush

_____

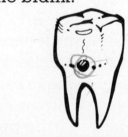

toothbrush   tooth decay
dental floss

_____

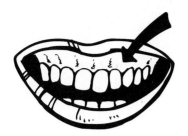

tongue   plaque
gums

_____

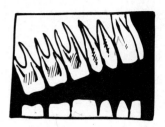

X-ray   mouthwash
plaque

_____

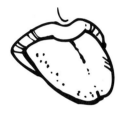

X-ray   gums
tongue

_____

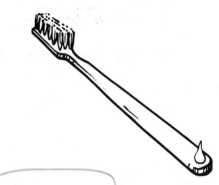

toothbrush   toothpaste
tooth decay

_____

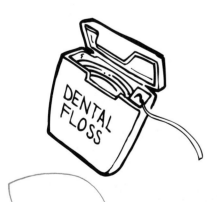

dental floss   toothpaste
tooth decay

_____

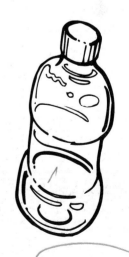

gums   mouthwash
dental floss

_____

Fill in the Blank

Fill in the blanks with the correct words from the list below.

toothbrush   toothpaste   gum disease
dental examinations   plaque   dental floss
tooth decay   tongue

Taking good care of your teeth and gums will save you pain and money. (1) _Plaque_ on your teeth can cause (2) _tooth decay_ in your teeth and (3) _gum disease_ in your gums. To help keep your teeth clean, you can put (4) _toothpaste_ on a (5) _toothbrush_ and brush them. Don't forget to brush your (6) _tongue_ too. To clean between your teeth, you can use (7) _dental floss_. Regular (8) _dental examinations_ from your dentist are important too.

Activity

Study conversations 1 and 2. Then complete conversation 3. Practice with a partner.

Conversation 1

Dentist: Do you brush your teeth at least twice a day?
Patient: Yes, I do.
Dentist: Do you floss your teeth?
Patient: Yes, I do.
Dentist: Do you have a dental examination every six months?
Patient: Yes, I do.

Conversation 2

Dentist: Do you brush your teeth at least twice a day?
Patient: No, I don't.
Dentist: Do you floss your teeth?
Patient: No, I don't.
Dentist: Do you have a dental examination every six months?
Patient: No, I don't.

Conversation 3

Dentist Do you brush your teeth at least twice a day?

Patient _yes I do_.

Dentist Do you floss your teeth?

Patient _NO I don't_.

Dentist Do you have a dental examination every six months?

Patient _sometime_.

Crossword Puzzle

Fill in the words from the word list below.

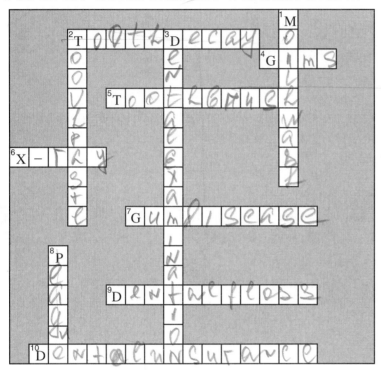

plaque
gums
toothbrush
tooth decay
X-ray
dental floss
dental
  examination
mouthwash
dental
  insurance
toothpaste
gum disease

ACROSS

2. brushing your teeth after meals helps prevent this
4. the pink tissue that holds your teeth in place
5. a brush used for cleaning teeth
6. a picture of your teeth
7. you have this if your gums are not healthy
9. a string used to clean between the teeth
10. a plan that pays for your dental care

DOWN

1. using this helps prevent bad breath
2. you put this on your tooth-brush
3. You should have a _____ _____ every year
8. a film built up on the teeth

Grammar 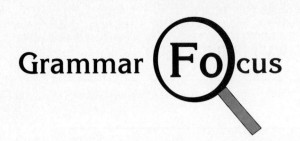cus

Present vs. Present Continuous

The present tense is used to express an action that goes on regularly or in general. The present continuous is used to describe an action that is going on right now.

For example: Present Tense

Theresa brushes her teeth every morning and evening. (Meaning: She brushes her teeth regularly.)

> (*Note:* For regular verbs in the third-person singular present tense, add an "s" at the end of the verb. For regular verbs which end in "ch," "sh," "j," "s," "x," and "z," add "es.")

For example: Present Continuous

Theresa is getting ready for bed. (She is doing it right now.)

> (*Note:* Form the present continuous by using the present tense form of the verb "to be" and adding "ing" to the infinitive form of the main verb.)

Fill in each blank with the correct form of the verb.

For example: She (brush) _____brushes_____ her teeth.
She <u>is</u> <u>brushing</u> her teeth.

1. The dentist (take) _____is taking_____ an X-ray of Theresa's teeth right now.

2. She (work) _____works_____ in a large office building every day.

3. Many people (go) _____go_____ away for the weekend because Monday is a holiday.

4. Theresa (clean) _____cleans_____ the plaque off her teeth every day.

5. Javier sometimes (wake up) _____Wakes up_____ with a toothache.

6. Yoko always (use) _____uses_____ dental floss.

What about you?

- ○ Do people use toothbrushes or something else to clean their teeth in your country?
- ○ Do people often go to the dentist in your country?
- ○ Do many people in your country have fillings?
- ○ Do people use mouthwash in your country?
- ○ Does the smell of people's mouths bother you?
- ○ Do you use dental floss?

=========== PRACTICE EXERCISES ===========

Interview

(pair activity)

Copy this chart, and then ask your partner the following questions and check off the appropriate box. Be prepared to report your findings to the class.

	Very often	Often	Sometimes	Seldom	Never
1. Do you ever have a toothache?	___	___	___	___	___
2. How often do you buy a new toothbrush?	___	___	___	___	___
3. Do you see a dentist?	___	___	___	___	___
4. Do you use dental floss?	___	___	___	___	___
5. Do you use a mouthwash?	___	___	___	___	___
6. Do people tell you that they like your smile?	___	___	___	___	___
7. Do you have X-rays taken of your teeth?	___	___	___	___	___
8. Do dentists charge too much money?	___	___	___	___	___
9. Do you sleep well at night?	___	___	___	___	___
10. Do you ever need to get a filling for a tooth?	___	___	___	___	___

Pronunciation Exercise
(pair activity)

Copy the following lists of words (Partner A's are listed here. Partner B's are in Appendix A, pages 220-221). Where it says "Listen and check" put a check mark by the word your partner pronounces. Where it says "Pronounce" say the word that is underlined, and your partner will put a check mark by that word. *Do not look at your partner's page.* When you are finished, correct your answers. If you don't know how to pronounce a word, ask the teacher.

PARTNER A

1. Listen and check:

   flows _____

   floss _____

   flaws _____

2. Pronounce:

   gum

   whom

   hum

3. Listen and check:

   tooth _____

   teeth _____

   tenth _____

4. Pronounce:

   tongue

   done

   tong

5. Listen and check:

   block _____

   black _____

   plaque _____

6. Pronounce:

   ache

   ace

   "h" (the letter)

7. Listen and check:

   moth _____

   month _____

   mouth _____

8. Pronounce:

   cold

   called

   cawed

9. Listen and check:

   comb _____

   come _____

   calm _____

10. Pronounce:

    cut

    cute

    caught

11. Listen and check:

racer	_____
resort	_____
razor	_____

12. Pronounce:

shower

sure

shore

Role Play

Act out the following situations (in groups of 3, 4, or 5). Be sure that everyone has something to say.

1. A dental insurance salesperson is trying to sell dental insurance to a person with a toothache. That person's friend says that dental insurance is a waste of money, so no matter what the insurance salesperson says, the friend argues against it.

2. Dudley Deadhead works in an office with three other people. Dudley has bad breath, and the other workers have to find a way to get him to do something about it.

3. A dentist is working on two patients. One patient has a cavity and needs a filling. This patient is very afraid of the dentist's drill. He/she thinks it is going to hurt. The other patient has no teeth at all and wants the dentist to give him/her false teeth. The dentist's helper keeps telling the dentist that the waiting room is full of other patients and that he/she needs to hurry up.

4. Mr. Tooth Decay and his good old friend Percy Plaque are trying to murder Ms. Tooth. Tuba Toothpaste and Denny Dental Floss are trying to save Ms. Tooth. They tell Ms. Tooth what she must do to save her own life.

5. A television commercial announcer for Smiley Toothpaste shows everyone the difference between a "Smiley" smile on one person and a "non-Smiley" smile on another. The "non-Smiley" person starts to beg for a tube of Smiley Toothpaste.

6. Two people are arguing about whether it is better to squeeze the toothpaste tube from the middle or from the end. A peacemaker comes in and settles the argument.

Nutrition

WORD LIST

Things

nutrition
health
weight
breakfast
disease
lunch
dinner
cafeteria
supermarket
restaurant
fat
cholesterol
cola
sugar
vitamins
minerals
menu

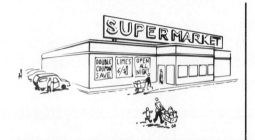
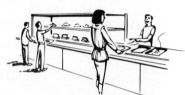
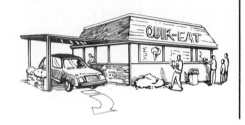
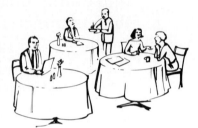

Actions

prepare

Descriptions

drive-in
overweight
sparingly

Tomas and Theresa know that good nutrition is important for good health. They need to eat the right foods to help prevent disease and control their weight. Their children need to eat the right foods to grow up strong and healthy.

Because Theresa and Tomas are both working, Tomas usually cooks dinner two or three times a week. At first he didn't like to cook, but now he thinks he can prepare some foods better than his wife. Theresa usually makes breakfast and helps Cathy pack her lunch for school. Mark eats his lunch in the school cafeteria.

Theresa usually buys the food for the family at the supermarket. Sometimes she buys a few things at smaller stores, but prices are best at the supermarket. When she shops she reads the nutrition labels and thinks about the six basic food groups:

1. Breads, cereals, rice, and pasta
2. Vegetables
3. Fruits
4. Milk, yogurt, and cheese
5. Meat, poultry, fish, dry beans, eggs, and nuts
6. Fats, oils, and sweets

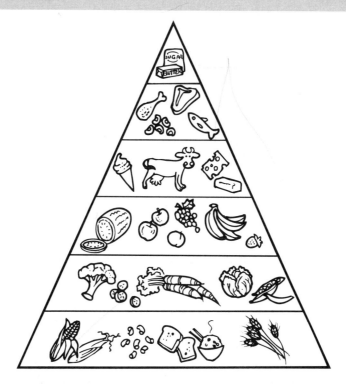

Today she is buying nonfat milk, cheese, and lowfat ice cream from the milk group. She knows that some foods with good nutrition, such as ice cream, are also high in fat or added sugar so she chooses reduced fat milk and ice cream. She's buying chicken, peanut butter, and pinto beans from the meat group. She's buying potatoes and carrots from the vegetable group. She's buying oranges and bananas from the fruit group. And she's buying whole wheat bread, noodles, and rice from the bread group.

Tomas doesn't like milk but he likes cheese. Mark and Cathy don't like carrots but they like potatoes. And Theresa doesn't like chicken but she likes fish. However, so that they can be healthy, all of them eat several servings from each group every day.

Comprehension Check

Circle the correct answer.

1. Who cooks dinner at the Santos' house?

    a. Tomas   b. Tomas and Theresa   c. Theresa

2. Theresa shops for food at _____.

    a. the supermarket   b. the cafeteria   c. school

3. Which food is not in the dairy group?

    a. peanut butter   b. ice cream   c. cheese

4. Which food is in the vegetable group?

    a. peanut butter   b. rice   c. carrots

5. Beans are in the meat group.

    a. true   b. false

6. Which food is not in the bread group?

    a. noodles   b. potatoes   c. rice

 # Cultural Note

Americans are always in a hurry. They want fast cars, fast service, fast answers, fast *everything*. But most of all, they want fast food. The drive-in hamburger stand is one of our most popular kinds of restaurants. But fast food is usually not healthful food. It is often high in fat, cholesterol, and sugar. And it is usually low in vitamins and minerals. For example, a hamburger and French fries are high in fat and cholesterol, which are leading causes of heart disease. Cola is all sugar and no nutrition. The only good news is that it's fast.

Most Americans eat more when they're in a hurry too. They eat without thinking about how much or how often they eat. Many Americans are overweight, which is very bad for their health.

The U.S. Department of Agriculture recommends the following daily number of servings from each food group.

1. Breads, cereals, rice, and pasta: 6-11 servings
2. Vegetables: 3-5 servings

3. Fruit: 2-4 servings
4. Milk, yogurt, and cheese: 2-3 servings
5. Meat, poultry, fish, dry beans, eggs, and nuts: 2-3 servings
6. Fats, oils, and sweets: eat sparingly

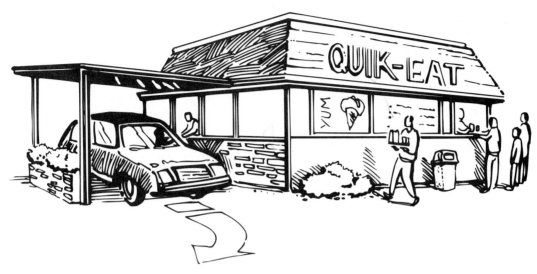

Fill in the Blank

Fill in the blanks with the correct words from the list below.

supermarket	prepare	fat	weight
cholesterol	restaurant	disease	vitamins
dinner	minerals	lunch	
nutrition	breakfast	health	

You should think about what you eat because (1) _Nutrition_ is important for good (2) _health_.
When you eat in a (3) _restaurant_ or shop at the (4) _lunch_ get foods that keep you healthy and help prevent (5) _disease_ and control (6) ~~choles~~ _weight_.
Foods that are low in (7) _cholesterol_ and (8) _fat_ are fruits and vegetables. These foods are also high in (9) _vitamins_ and (10) _minerals_ and are easy to (11) _prepare_. Fruits and vegetables are good choices for (12) _breakfast_ in the morning, (13) _for lunch_ in the middle of the day, and (14) _for dinner_ in the evening.

Activity 1

Put the words from the list below in the proper food group. Work with a partner.

tomatoes	chicken	eggs	strawberries
hamburgers	ice cream	bananas	oatmeal
milk	bread	rolls	shrimp
broccoli	pork chops	noodles	yogurt

Milk, Yogurt, & Cheese Group

_____

_____

_____

_____

Meat, Poultry, Fish, Dry Beans, and Eggs Group

_____

_____

_____

_____

Vegetable Group

_____

_____

_____

_____

Fruit Group

_____

_____

_____

_____

Bread, Cereal, Rice, and Pasta Group

_____

_____

_____

_____

Activity 2

Using the list of foods in Activity 1, make a menu for breakfast, lunch, and dinner. Work with a partner.

Breakfast _____ _____ _____ _____

Lunch _____ _____ _____ _____

Dinner _____ _____ _____ _____

Activity 3

In groups of 3 to 4 students, number the following statements in order of importance. Present your answers to the class.

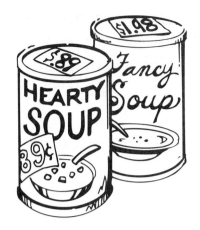

When I buy food . . .

____ price is very important.

____ good nutrition is more important than price or taste

____ good taste is more important than low price.

Grammar 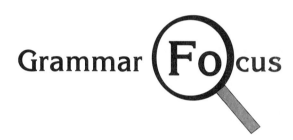 cus

The use of "usually"

The word "usually" is used to describe something that happens most of the time. Notice that "usually" comes just before the verb.

> *For example:* Theresa usually makes breakfast. (Meaning: Most of the time Theresa makes breakfast.)

Rewrite the sentences below using the word "usually."

> *For example:* Most of the time Pedro goes to the movies on Saturday.
> Pedro usually goes to the movies on Saturday.

1. Most of the time I eat foods from the five main food groups.
   I _____.

2. Most of the time Theresa rides her bicycle to the supermarket.
   Theresa _____.

3. Tomas almost always cooks dinner two or three times a week.
   Tomas_____.

4. Most of the time she eats lunch in the school cafeteria.
   She _____.

5. They nearly always eat cereal, toast, and fruit for breakfast.
   They _____.

What about you?

○ Do you eat foods every day from the six main food groups?
○ Do you eat too much or too little food?
○ Do you eat canned food?
○ Do you eat frozen food?
○ Do you like American food?
○ When you're in a hurry, do you eat more food or different food?

═══ PRACTICE EXERCISES ═══

Find Someone in the Class Who . . .

1. knows the six food groups and can name them _____
2. is on a diet _____
3. had cereal for breakfast _____
4. doesn't usually eat breakfast _____
5. doesn't like ice cream _____
6. gets up in the middle of the night and raids the refrigerator _____
7. likes to eat several small meals a day instead of three regular ones _____
8. likes chocolate _____
9. knows his/her cholesterol count _____
10. never cooks _____
11. eats at a fast food restaurant at least once a week _____
12. wants to gain weight _____
13. likes to cook _____
14. takes a packed lunch to school or work _____
15. buys lunch every day _____
16. hates to go grocery shopping _____
17. likes lima beans _____
18. is a vegetarian _____
19. takes vitamin pills _____
20. never drinks cola _____

Art Project

(groups of 4 or 5)

For this project you will need one large piece of cardboard (at least 18" x 18") per group, scissors, and glue. Bring magazines and grocery store advertisements to class. Divide the cardboard into six equal sections and label each one a different food group. From the advertisements (preferably color ones), cut out all the examples you can find for each of the six food groups. Form a collage by gluing the food together in the appropriate section. Don't forget to label every food. Someone admiring your artwork may want to know the name of something.

Conversation

(pair activity)

Partner A will start the following conversation (question 1). Partner B must then decide which response (question 2, a or b) is appropriate. Partner A will then respond with the appropriate response (question 3, a or b) to Partner B, and so on. The conversation will not make sense unless the right choices are made.

PARTNER A

1. Would you like to grab something quick to eat in this fast food restaurant?

3. a. You could order the chicken salad with diet dressing. Does that sound good?

   b. They have some delicious ice cream. Do you want two scoops or three?

5. a. I never eat more than three. Do you want ketchup on your French fries?

   b. A bacon cheeseburger, French fries, chocolate milkshake, and ice cream. Do you think that's a good idea?

PARTNER B

2. a. Sure, I love candlelit dinners and white tablecloths. Do they serve gourmet food?

   b. OK, but I'm on a diet. Do they have any food that's not fattening?

4. a. That will be perfect. What are you going to have?

   b. Oh, I think I will. What do you want for dessert?

6. a. Why not? We should always eat a healthy, well-balanced meal.

   b. I think that maybe you should find out your cholesterol count from your doctor!

4 Exercise and Weight Control

WORD LIST

Things
exercise
diet
physical
examination
energy
stairs
elevator
habit
dessert
meal
heart rate
heart
lungs
height

Descriptions
annual

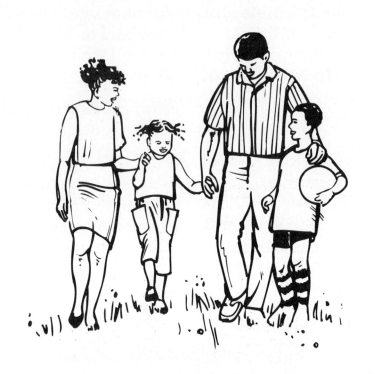

Theresa and her family have a good diet of healthful foods. But we all need good food *and* exercise for good health.

Yesterday Theresa went for her annual physical examination. Her doctor said she needs to lose ten pounds. She often feels tired. The doctor said she needs to exercise.

Theresa told the doctor, "I don't have time to exercise. I'm too busy with my job, my family, and the house." But he explained to her that exercise will make her feel better. She'll have more energy.

Now she's thinking, "I can use the stairs instead of the elevator at work. When I go to work, I can walk to a bus stop farther from my house. I can ride my bicycle to the store if I only need a few things. I can walk with my family or a friend instead of sitting down to watch television or drink coffee."

But Theresa knows it's important to begin slowly. And she knows she needs to make exercise a habit if she wants to feel better and look better. She also wants the new dress she's going to buy when she loses the ten pounds. This morning Theresa is leaving for the supermarket on her bicycle. Her 14 year-old son, Mark, is saying, "My mom on a bicycle! I don't believe it!"

Comprehension Check

Circle the correct answer.

1. Theresa's family has a good diet.

   a. true   b. false

2. Where did Theresa go yesterday?

   a. to the supermarket   b. to work   c. to the doctor

3. What does Theresa need to do?

   a. have a physical examination   b. rest   c. lose ten pounds

4. Exercise will make Theresa tired.

   a. true   b. false

5. What can Theresa do for exercise?

   a. use the stairs at work   b. watch television   c. ride the bus

6. What does Theresa want?

   a. a bicycle   b. a new dress   c. a television

Cultural Note

Many Americans eat too much. They may eat foods from all the food groups, but add too much bread or dessert. And they may eat between meals.

Exercise is important in weight control, but it makes you feel good too. It makes all parts of your body work better. It gives you more energy and makes you less tired because your heart rate is lower.

To keep your heart and lungs healthy, and your weight right, exercise for at least 30 minutes three times a week.

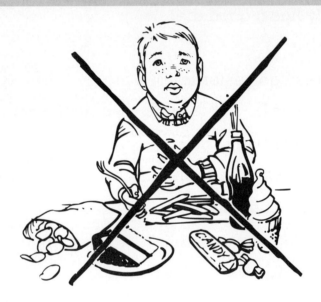

Vocabulary Builder

Circle the correct word and write the word in the blank.

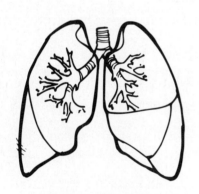

heart   lungs
heart rate

_____

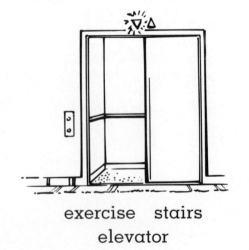

exercise   stairs
elevator

_____

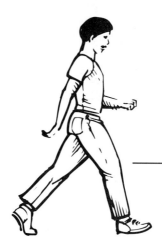

exercise   stairs
elevator

_____

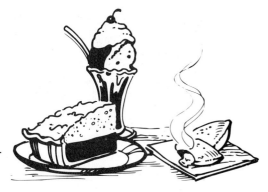

dessert   meal
height

_____

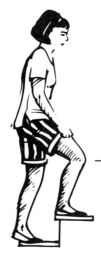

energy   heart rate
stairs

_____

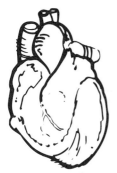

exercise   heart
stairs

_____

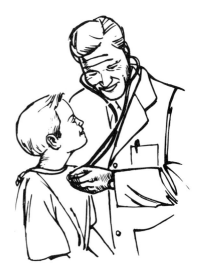

physical examination
habit   annual

_____

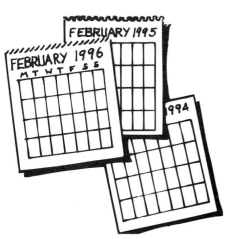

exercise   annual
height

_____

Grammar 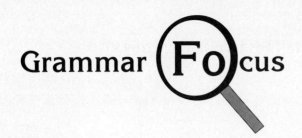cus

Use of "can"

The word "can" is used to show ability. Notice that in sentences the word "can" comes just before the verb. In questions the word "can" precedes the subject.

For example: Heidi can speak English. (Meaning: Heidi has the ability to speak English.) *or*
Can Heidi speak English? (Meaning: Does Heidi have the ability to speak English?)

The use of "can" may also show intention.

For example: I can come to your house for dinner on Saturday)
(Meaning: I will come to your house on Saturday.

Write sentences or questions using "can."

For example: Aura has the ability to swim.
<u>Aura</u> <u>can</u> <u>swim.</u>

1. Theresa has the ability to ride a bicycle.

   _____.

2. Tomas has the ability to cook.

   _____.

3. Theresa intends to walk with her family.

   _____.

4. Does Daniel have the ability to speak English?

   _____.

5. Does Theresa intend to use the stairs?

   _____.

What about you?
   ◯ Are you the right weight for your height?
   ◯ Do you have energy to get through the day?

❍ How often do you exercise?

❍ What can you change in your life to get more exercise?

PRACTICE EXERCISES

Interview
(pair activity)

Ask your partner the following questions about his/her physical exercise activity. Then come up with three suggestions for your partner to improve his/her exercise program.

1. Do you think you get enough exercise? **Yes** _____ **No** _____

2. Do you ride a bicycle? **Yes** _____ **No** _____

3. Do you think you walk a lot? **Yes** _____ **No** _____

   If yes, when and where? _____

   _____.

   _____.

4. Do you get tired at a certain time of day? **Yes** _____ **No** _____
   If yes, what time, usually? _____

5. How often do you exercise? _____

   _____

6. What kind of exercise do you like most? _____

   _____

7. What kind of exercise do you not like? _____

   _____

8. What time of day is the best time for you to exercise? _____

   _____

9. When you can choose between stairs and
   an elevator, which one do you take? **Stairs** _____ **Elevator** _____

10. Do you think exercise gives you more
    energy? **Yes** _____ **No** _____

Now write three **specific** suggestions for your partner to improve his/her exercise program:

1. My partner should _____

2. My partner should _____

3. My partner should _____

Lesson 4   Exercise and Weight Control   **33**

Information Gaps

(pair activity; past tense, asking questions)

Ask your partner for the information for your blank boxes. Use the conversation below. Write the information in your boxes. Partner B's chart is in Appendix A, page 221. *Do not look at your partner's page.*

PARTNER A

A: What did _____ do yesterday at _____?

B: He/she_____. (Be sure to fill in the correct past tense.)

Name	6:30 A.M.	4:30 P.M.	8:30 P.M.
Jim Nasium	(go) _____ jogging		
Ann Exercise		(do) _____ aerobics	(take) _____ a walk
Dan D. Dancer	(jump) _____ rope		(do) _____ the lambada
C. Potato		(eat) _____ 2 bags of potato chips & (watch) _____ TV	

Continuous Line Drill

(past tense reinforcement drill)

Your teacher will tell half of your class to each write one of the following verbs on a piece of paper. Then those people will form an outside circle. The other half of the class will form an inside circle facing the outside circle. When the teacher says "Start" the people on the inside will move from one outside person to the next. They must both pronounce and spell the *past tense* of each verb. When everyone has gone around twice, the inside circle will take the cards of the outside circle, and the same process will go on the other way around.

For example: <u>On the paper</u>   <u>Answer</u>

go (present tense)   **went** (past tense)

go	see	say	run
ride	eat	have	feel
tell	think	sit	drink
take	know	begin	leave

Let's Play Charades
(practice in asking questions)

The following exercise activities will be written out on separate pieces of paper. The class will be divided into two teams. One person from each team will take turns acting out the exercise activity written on the piece of paper which the teacher will hand out. In order to win a point, a member of that person's team must identify the activity *and* must phrase the question correctly.

For example: "Are you jogging?"

riding a bicycle	aerobics
walking	lifting weights
playing tennis	playing baseball
playing golf	playing American football
playing soccer	bowling
jumping hurdles	doing jumping jacks
jumping rope	jumping on a trampoline
climbing stairs	roller skating
dancing	skiing
ice skating	operating TV remote control
doing situps	(for the couch potato in the
swimming	group)

5

Taking Your Temperature

WORD LIST

Things

temperature
thermometer
receptionist
county hospital
symptoms
headache
sore throat
oral temperature
rectal temperature
fluids

Actions

shaking
reading

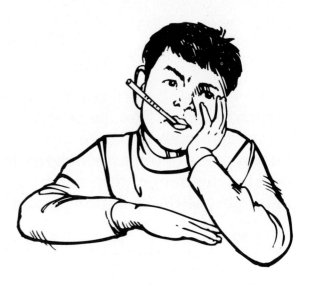

Descriptions

Fahrenheit
Celsius

normal
accurate

It's Monday morning. Mark didn't sleep well at all last night. He aches all over, and he feels very warm. Ah! Some cold orange juice tastes good.

Theresa wants to take his temperature in his mouth, but she needs to wait five or ten minutes because the cold juice changes Mark's temperature. She's waiting and shaking the thermometer so the temperature reading drops below 98.6 degrees Fahrenheit. Mark doesn't want his mother to take his temperature. He says he can do it himself.

At last, Mark's mother puts the thermometer all the way in under his tongue. "Close your mouth," she tells him, "and lie still." Then she looks at her watch. She leaves the thermometer in place for three minutes.

When she removes the thermometer she reads Mark's temperature. It's 103 degrees Fahrenheit! That's almost five degrees above the normal 98.6 degrees. It's time to visit the doctor.

Theresa is calling the county hospital.

Theresa: My son's temperature is 103 degrees. He needs to see a doctor.

Receptionist: What other symptoms does he have?

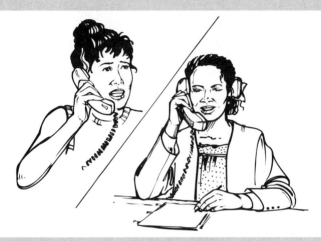

Theresa: He has a bad headache and a sore throat.

Receptionist: Can he come in at 10 o'clock?

Theresa: Yes. I'll have to leave work to drive him. Thank you.

Receptionist: If you have insurance, bring your card.

Comprehension Check

Circle the correct answer.

1. How does Mark feel?

   a. achy   b. well   c. hungry

2. What does Theresa want to do?

   a. give Mark some juice   b. wait five or ten minutes

   c. take Mark's temperature

3. How long does she leave the thermometer in Mark's mouth?

   a. five minutes   b. three minutes   c. one minute

4. Who gives Mark an appointment at the hospital?

   a. a receptionist   b. a doctor   c. a patient

Cultural Note

When taking an oral temperature is not possible, such as with small children and people who are sleeping, take a rectal temperature. Use an oral thermometer for an oral temperature and a rectal thermometer for a rectal temperature. The normal oral temperature is 98.6 degrees Fahrenheit and the normal rectal temperature, which is more accurate, is 99.6 degrees. These are morning temperatures. Evening temperatures are usually one degree higher.

It's important to know if you or your child has a temperature. *Children should not go to school if they have a temperature.* They might make other children sick and they need to rest at home.

Anyone who has a temperature should stay away from other people, drink lots of fluids, and sleep as much as possible.

How to Convert Temperatures

If you want to change degrees Celsius to degrees

Fahrenheit: C = Celsius F = Fahrenheit

$$F = \frac{9}{5} C + 32$$

For example: C = 38

38 x 9 = 342 ÷ 5 = 68.4 + 32 = 100.4 degrees F

If you want to change degrees Fahrenheit to degrees Celsius:

C = Celsius F = Fahrenheit $F = \frac{5}{9} (F - 32)$

For example: F = 103

103 - 32 = 71 x 5 = 355 ÷ 9 = 39.4 degrees C

Temperature Conversion

Can you change these temperatures?

Change from Celsius to Fahrenheit:	Change from Fahrenheit to Celsius:
35 degrees _____	105 degrees _____
28 degrees _____	80 degrees _____
20 degrees _____	65 degrees _____

Crossword Puzzle

Fill in the words from the word list below.

Word list:
thermometer
receptionist
accurate
Fahrenheit
temperature
 reading
normal
fluid
sore throat
headache
Celsius
symptoms
shaking
hospital

(Grid with numbered cells: 1T, 2R, 3F, 4R, 5F, 6A, 7H, 8T, 9S, 10H, 11N, 12S, 13C, 14S)

ACROSS

1. an instrument used to take temperature
6. correct
8. how hot or cold it is
11. usual
12. it is hard to swallow when you have this
13. a way of reading temperature: Fahrenheit or _____
14. moving quickly back and forth

DOWN

2. the person who first greets you
3. A way of reading temperature: Celsius or _____
4. the temperature _____ is 100.6 degrees F
5. juice, water, and tea are examples of this
7. pain in the head
9. a sore throat, a fever, and a headache are _____ of the flu
10. a place where people get medical treatment

Grammar 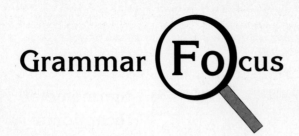cus

Present Tense

The present tense is used to express an action that goes on in general.

> *For example:* Orange juice tastes good.

> (*Note:* For regular verbs in the third-person singular present tense, add an "s" at the end of the verb. For regular verbs that end in "ch," "sh," "j," "s," [x," and "z," add "es.")

Fill in the correct present tense form of the verb in the following sentences.

> *For example:* Plaque (cause) _____ gum disease.
> Plaque <u>causes</u> gum disease.

1. Theresa (want) _____ to take Mark's temperature.

2. It (be) _____ Monday morning.

3. I (leave) _____ the thermometer in place for three minutes.

4. He (need) _____ to see a doctor.

5. He (have) _____ a bad headache and a sore throat.

6. We (want) _____ you to see a doctor.

What about you?

○ Do you stay in bed when you have a temperature?

○ If you have children, do you keep them home when they have a temperature?

PRACTICE EXERCISES

Choral Reading: Song
(group activity)

As a class, read or sing to the tune of "It's Raining, It's Pouring." The first time, read all the words. The second time, instead of saying the first bold, italicized word, act it out instead. The third time through, act out the first two bold, italicized words instead of saying them, and so on.

It's raining, it's pouring
The old man is *snoring.*
He went to bed with a bump on his head
And couldn't get up in the morning.
Came down with *the chills*
So he *took some pills*
But he got more sick without warning.

First he got a *headache*
And then he got a *cough.*
And then he had a *runny nose*
He wished he could turn off.

Next he got a *stomachache*
And then a *bad sore throat*
He couldn't even *lift his head*
Or keep his mind afloat.

His appetite had disappeared
He couldn't *eat* at all.
But when he got *an itchy rash*
The doctor he did call.

The doctor *shook his finger*
And said, "You're very ill.
But you may still be sicker yet
When you receive my bill."

Information Gaps

(pair activity; past tense, asking questions)

Ask your partner for the information for your blank boxes. Use the conversation below. Write the information in your boxes. Partner B's chart is in Appendix A, page 222. *Do not look at your partner's page*

PARTNER A

A: What is _____'s temperature?

B: His/her temperature is _____ degrees.

A: What are his/her other symptoms?

B: He/she has _____.

Name	Temperature	Symptom	Symptom
Ann Teabody	101.6		a sore throat
Mike Robe		no appetite	
Scarlet O'Fever	103.4	a rash	
Rob Itussin			a stomachache

Tag Questions

(pair activity)

Take one part in the following dialogue, and fill in the proper words for the tag questions.

For example: A: Look at Mark. He looks so tired this morning.

B: He didn't sleep very well last night, <u>did he</u> ?

A: Mark says he aches all over and feels very warm.

B: He has a fever, _____ _____? Give him some cold orange juice.

A: O.K. I want to take his temperature, but if I give him cold juice, I need to wait five or ten minutes, _____ _____?

B: Yes, because the juice will change his temperature. You're going to shake the thermometer before you give it to him,_____ _____?

A: Oh, yes. I almost forgot. The temperature needs to be below 98.6 degrees before I put it under his tongue, _____ _____?

B: Yes, and then you need to keep the thermometer under his tongue for three minutes.

(Later)

A: 103 degrees! That's almost five degrees above normal, _____ _____?

B: Yes, it is. You're going to call the doctor, _____ _____?

A: Yes. The phone number for the county hospital is in the phone book, _____ _____?

B: I think so. You don't have it written in your address book, _____ _____?

A. No, but that's a good idea for the future. Let's see. I need to tell the doctor about his other symptoms, _____ _____?

B: Yes. He has a bad headache, _____ _____?

A: And a sore throat, too. I hope the doctor will see him soon. You don't need the car today, _____ _____?

B: No, you take it. I hope Mark feels better soon.

6 Prescription and Nonprescription Drugs

WORD LIST

Things
flu
fever
prescription
antibiotic
aspirin
pharmacy
dosage
generic form
ingredients
brand
medicine

Descriptions
nonprescription
well

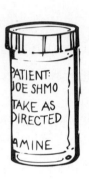

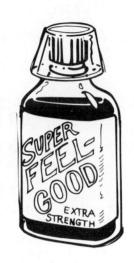

It's Monday afternoon, but Mark isn't at school. He's home in bed with the flu. He feels awful. He has a headache, a sore throat, and a fever.

His mother drove him to the doctor at the county hospital this morning. The doctor gave him a prescription for an antibiotic. He told Mark to take it every day until he finishes it, even if he feels O.K.

Theresa filled the prescription at the pharmacy, and also bought some aspirin, which is a nonprescription drug. This morning Mark's temperature was 103 degrees Fahrenheit. Now he's taking aspirin for his fever and headache—two tablets every four hours. This is an adult dosage because he's more than 12 years old.

But he needs more than aspirin and an antibiotic to get well. He needs lots of rest and sleep. He doesn't mind staying home from school to rest, but on Friday night he wants to go out to the movies with his friends.

Comprehension Check

Circle the correct answer.

1. Is Mark at school today?

   a. Yes, he is.   b. No, he isn't.

2. Mark has a _____.

   a. stomachache   b. fever   c. earache

3. An antibiotic is a prescription drug.

   a. true   b. false

4. For his fever and headache Mark is taking _____.

   a. aspirin   b. an antibiotic   c. a prescription drug

 Cultural Note

   You can usually save money when you buy the generic form of a drug. Prescription and nonprescription drugs come in generic form. When the doctor writes a prescription for you, ask him for the generic form. When you buy a nonprescription drug, look at the price and look at the ingredients. One brand of aspirin, for example, may cost more than another, but the ingredients may be the same, so the medicine is the same.

   Don't share your prescription with another person. Medicine that is good for you may not be good for someone else even if the symptoms are the same. A doctor must decide what medicine a person should take.

   Also, give children a child's dosage of nonprescription drugs. And don't give any of your drugs to pets.

Crossword Puzzle

Fill in the words from the word list below.

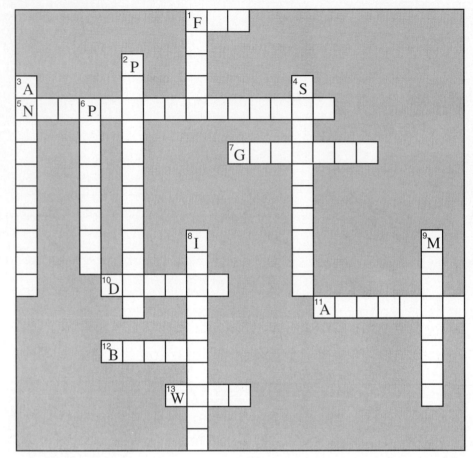

ingredient
well
prescription
medicine
nonprescription
aspirin
antibiotic
brand
flu
dosage
sore throat
generic
pharmacy
fever

ACROSS

1. what you have when you feel sick all over
5. a drug you can buy at the store without a doctor's order
7. the medical name for a drug (not the brand name)
10. the amount of medicine you should take
11. a common drug you take for a fever
12. "Tylenol" is the _____ name for a drug.
13. when you're sick people say, "Get _____ soon!"

DOWN

1. temperature above 98.6 degrees Fahrenheit
2. a drug only a doctor can give you
3. a drug to get rid of an infection
4. pain in your throat
6. a store where you buy medicine
8. some medicines have more than one _____
9. something you take to get well

Fill in the Blank

Fill in the blanks with the correct words from the list below.

brands	generic form	fever	antibiotic
medicine	prescription	ingredients	flu
aspirin	pharmacy		

It's no fun to be sick, but when the thermometer says you have
a (1) _____, (2) _____ can help.
When you have the (3) _____ the doctor can write
you a (4) _____ for an (5) _____ to
help you get well. When the doctor writes you a prescription,
take it to a (6) _____. At the pharmacy, you can
save money when you buy the (7) _____
_____ of the (8) _____ you need.
Generic drugs often come in many (9) _____, but
they all have the same (10) _____.

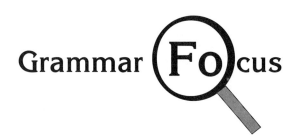

Grammar Focus

Present Continuous

The present continuous is used to describe an action that is going on right now. Form the present continuous by using the present tense form of the verb "to be" and adding "ing" to the infinitive form of the main verb.

For example: Mark <u>is</u> tak<u>ing</u> his medicine.

   (*Note:* If the infinitive form of the verb ends in a silent "e", drop the "e" before adding "ing.")

Change the following sentences from the present tense to the present continuous by filling in the blanks.

For example: Mark goes to school every day. (present)
        Mark <u>is</u> <u>going</u> to school. (present continous)

1. Mark takes antibiotics for his flu. Mark _____ _____ antibiotics for his flu.

2. He stays home from school when he is sick. He _____ _____ home from school.

3. He takes aspirin for his fever. Now he _____ _____ aspirin for his fever.

4. The doctor gives him a prescription. The doctor _____ _____ him a prescription.

5. It's Friday night. He and his friends go to the movies every Friday night. He and his friends _____ _____ to the movies.

6. He gets lots of sleep and rest. He _____ _____ lots of sleep and rest today.

7. Mark's mother fills the prescription. Mark's mother _____ _____ the prescription.

8. Theresa buys aspirin for her family. Theresa _____ _____ aspirin.

What about you?

○ Do you buy generic drugs to save money?
○ Do you share your drugs with any other person?

—— PRACTICE EXERCISES ——

Past Tense

(pair or individual activity)

Change the verbs in the following sentences into the past tense.

For example: It (be) _____**was**_____ Monday morning. Mark (feel) _____**felt**_____ awful.

This morning Mark (**1. be**) _____ at home in bed. He (**2. have**) _____ a headache, a sore throat, and a fever. His mother (**3. drive**) _____ him to the doctor's office. The doctor (**4. give**) _____ him a prescription for an antibiotic. He (**5. tell**) _____ Mark to take it every day.

His mother (**6. get**) _____ the prescription filled at the pharmacy. She (**7. know**) _____ that she (**8. can**) _____ save money by buying the generic form of the drug. That is why she had asked the doctor to write the generic form on the prescription. She also (**9. buy**) _____ some aspirin for Mark. By comparing the different prices and looking at the ingredients in the aspirin bottles, she (**10. find**) _____ the best price for the aspirin.

Before giving Mark the medicine, his mother (**11. study**) _____ the dosage instructions carefully. She (**12. do**) _____ not want to give him too much or too little. She (**13. put**) _____ the medicine in a safe place after she (**14. give**) _____ it to Mark so that no one else would use it. She (**15. know**) _____ that prescription drugs are to be used only by the person whose name is on the bottle.

Proper Dosages

(pair activity)

Study the medicine bottle. You and your partner will take turns presenting the problem and choosing the correct solution from answers a, b, and c.

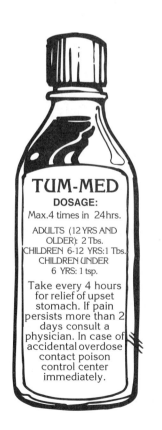

TUM-MED
DOSAGE:
Max.4 times in 24hrs.

ADULTS (12 YRS AND OLDER): 2 Tbs.
CHILDREN 6-12 YRS:1 Tbs.
CHILDREN UNDER 6 YRS: 1 tsp.

Take every 4 hours for relief of upset stomach. If pain persists more than 2 days consult a physician. In case of accidental overdose contact poison control center immediately.

PARTNER A

1. Ana is nine years old today. She just woke up with a stomachache.

2. a. He should take 2 tablespoonfuls of TUM-MED immediately.

    b. He should call his doctor.

    c. He should contact a poison control center.

3. It's Christmas Eve. Four-year-old Billy has a tummyache from eating too many candy canes.

4. a. It's O.K. because the medicine has already expired.

   b. Someone should call the poison control center immediately.

   c. She should wait 24 hours before she drinks any more.

5. It's July 5th. Eleven-year-old Julia ate too much at the picnic yesterday. She took 1 tablespoon of TUM-MED last night at 7:00 p.m., another at midnight, another at 6:00 a.m. this morning, and another at noon. Now it is 3:00 p.m. and she wants another tablespoon of TUM-MED.

6. a. He should take two teaspoons of TUM-MED.

   b. He should take two tablespoons of TUM-MED.

   c. He should not take this medicine because it has expired.

PARTNER B

1. a. She should take one tablespoonful of TUM-MED.

   b. She should take one teaspoonful of TUM-MED.

   c. She should take two teaspoonfuls of TUM-MED.

2. Twenty-five-year old Samuel has had a stomachache for three days.

3. a. He should take one teaspoonful of TUM-MED.

   b. He should not take this medicine because he's too young.

   c. Someone should call the poison control center immediately.

4. Grandma Abuelita thought that TUM-MED was a strawberry milkshake and she just drank a whole glassful.

5. a. She can have another tablespoon of TUM-MED now.

   b. She can have one teaspoon of TUM-MED now and one more teaspoon in 4 hours.

   c. She will have to wait until 7:00 tonight before she takes any more.

6. Nineteen-year-old Jaime has a stomachache from too much partying the night before.

Dice Game
(group activity)

Taking turns, roll a die and move the number of spaces shown. If you land on an empty square, stay there and wait for your next turn. If you land on a square with a sentence, say whether it is correct or wrong. If it is wrong, correct it. If you are right, move ahead two squares. If you are wrong, move back two squares.

FINISH 50	"Dosage" means "amount." 49	Prescriptions may be shared with others. 48	47	You wash your body with a razor. 46
41	You shave with a nail clipper. 42	43	You use dental floss to remove plaque between teeth. 44	45
There are two basic food groups. 40	Beef belongs to the bread and cereal food group. 39	38	37	Fast foods are the healthiest foods. 36
31	A normal temperature is 96.8 degrees. 32	33	34	Children should go to school with a fever. 35
30	A thermometer should stay under the tongue.for 2o seconds 29	28	27	Only a doctor can give a prescription. 26
You can save money by buying generic drugs 21	22	23	Antibiotics are prescription drugs. 24	25
20	You can get a prescription filled at a restaurant. 19	18	You brush your teeth after you go to bed. 17	16
You wash your hair with toothpaste 11	12	An X-ray is a prescription drug. 13	14	You brush your teeth with tooth decay. 15
10	Fats do not belong to any of the food groups. 9	Noodles belong to the milk group. 8	7	A bacon cheeseburger is low in cholesterol. 6
START 1	Today I **make**; yesterday I **maked**. 2	Today I **feel**; yesterday I **feeled**. 3	4	Today I **think**; yesterday I **thank**. 5

7 First Aid

WORD LIST

Things

first aid
picnic
barbecue
water fountain
napkin
ice chest
bleeding
bandage
bruise
swelling
nosebleed
nostrils
injuries
illness
wound
skin
poisoning
broken bone
unconsciousness

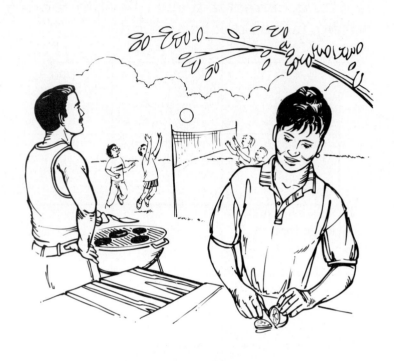

Actions

burn
press
pinch
lift
pat

Descriptions

careful
minor
serious

It's a beautiful summer day and the Santos Family is at the park for a picnic. Everyone is having a good time, but they should all be more careful.

Tomas is cooking hamburgers on the barbecue and he burns his hand. It's not a serious burn, but it hurts. He goes to the water fountain and runs cold water on it. Then he dips a napkin in the ice chest with the cold drinks and puts it on the burn. Ahhh, that feels better. Oh no! Now the hamburgers are burning!

Theresa is slicing tomatoes to put on the hamburgers and cuts her finger with the knife. She grabs a napkin and presses it against the cut to stop the bleeding. She holds her finger up as she goes to the restroom and washes the cut with soap and water. She dries the cut with a clean paper towel and puts a bandage on the cut.

Mark is playing volleyball with some other people in the park and falls and bruises his elbow. He puts some ice from the ice chest in a plastic bag and puts it on the bruise to keep the swelling down, but he wants to go back and play volleyball.

Cathy is watching the volleyball game. She's standing too close so the ball hits her nose and she gets a nosebleed. One of the volleyball players calls to Theresa and tells Cathy to sit down on a bench, lean forward, and pinch her nostrils closed until the bleeding stops.

What a day! They should all be more careful! But they had a good time anyway. Even the burned hamburgers tasted good!

Comprehension Check

Circle the correct answer.

1. What season is it?

   a. summer   b. spring   c. fall

2. The Santos family is having a _____.

   a. park   b. picnic   c. careful

3. What does Tomas do?

   a. He burns his hand.   b. He bruises his elbow.

   c. He cuts his finger.

4. What does Theresa do?

   a. She gets a nosebleed.   b. She burns her hand.

   c. She cuts her finger.

5. Mark _____ his elbow.

   a. cuts   b. burns   c. bruises

6. Cathy gets a _____.

   a. cut   b. nosebleed   c. burn

First Aid Procedures

For more serious injuries: Minor injuries or illness can become serious if no one gives first aid. Even if a person needs to go quickly to a doctor, you can help in the first few minutes. For example:

○ **For serious bleeding**—Do not wash the wound. Press on it with a clean bandage, cloth, or towel. Lift the wound above the heart if possible. Let a doctor or other medical worker take off the bandage and wash the wound.

○ **For serious burns**—If the burn isn't too large, wash it in cold water. Pat it dry and cover it with a clean bandage if the skin is open. Give aspirin for pain. See a doctor for large or deep burns.

○ **For poisoning**—Children sometimes eat or drink things they shouldn't. Look for a bottle nearby so you know what poison it is. Do not give the person anything to eat or drink. Call the Poison Control Center in your city. If he is unconscious, call 911.

○ **For broken bones**—Do not touch or move the bones. If there are wounds too, do not wash them, but stop the bleeding if necessary. Call 911 or go to a hospital emergency room.

○ **For unconsciousness**—If you can't wake a person up after an injury or the beginning of an illness, call 911.

○ **For gunshot wounds**—DO NOT remove metal objects from the wound. Follow the treatment for serious bleeding.

○ **For shock**—Make the person lie down with the feet a little higher than the head. Keep him/her warm. Do not give fluids. Call 911.

For more information on how you can help someone in an emergency, call the American Red Cross office in your city.

Word Groups

Cross out the word that does not belong.

1. napkin   nosebleed   barbeque   ice chest
2. burn   press   serious   lift
3. careful   broken bone   bruise   nosebleed
4. wound   minor   bleeding   poisoning

Vocabulary Builder

Circle the correct word and write the word in the blank.

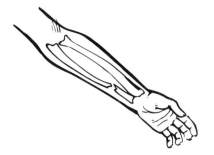

wound   nostrils
broken bone

_____

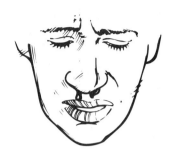

unconsciousness   burn
nosebleed

_____

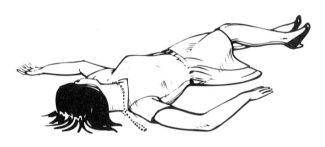

bandage   unconsciousness
swelling

_____

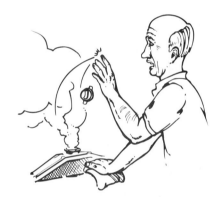

burn   bleeding
broken bone

_____

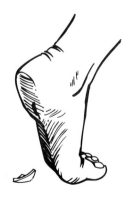

bruise   wound
poisoning

_____

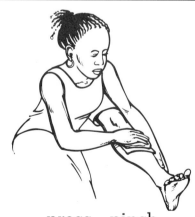

press   pinch
lift

_____

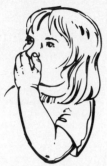

lift   pinch
pat

_____

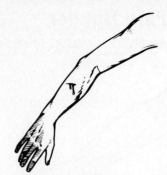

unconsciousness   bleeding
broken bone

_____

Matching

Match the word with the correct first aid response.

1. ____ bruise
2. ____ poisoning
3. ____ nosebleed
4. ____ burn

5. ____ broken bones
6. ____ bleeding
7. ____ unconsciousness

8. ____ shock

a. press with a clean bandage
b. call 911
c. do not touch or move them
d. lean forward and pinch nostrils
e. wash with cold water
f. put ice on this
g. find the bottle and call the Poison Control Center
h. make the person lie down

Grammar 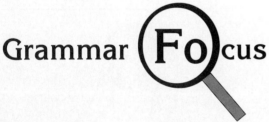 cus

Use of "but"

Use the word "but" after a statement when you want to make another statement that seems opposite.

For example: It's not a serious burn, but it hurts.

Choose a statement from the list to complete the following sentences:

For example: She likes dogs, but _____.
              She likes dogs, but she doesn't like cats.

she likes hot dogs
he put ice on it to stop the
  swelling
they had a good time
I can learn it

he's in bed with the flu
she pressed with a napkin to stop
  the bleeding
they tasted good
they should all be more careful

1. Everyone is having a good time, but _____

   _____.

2. They all got hurt, but _____

   _____.

3. She cut herself, but _____

   _____.

4. She doesn't like hamburgers, but _____

   _____.

5. Mark wants to go to the movies, but _____

   _____.

6. The hamburgers were burned, but _____

   _____.

7. Mark bruised his elbow, but _____

   _____.

8. English is difficult, but _____

   _____.

What about you?

   ○ Have you ever used first aid to help someone? What did you
     do?
   ○ Have you ever needed first aid? What happened?

PRACTICE EXERCISES

Pronunciation Exercise

(pair activity)

Copy the following lists of words (Partner A's are listed here. Partner B's are in Appendix A, pages 223-224). Where it says "Listen and check" put a check by the word your partner pronounces. Where it says "Pronounce" say the word that is underlined, and your partner will put a check mark by that word. *Do not look at your partner's page.* When you are finished, correct your answers. If you don't know how to pronounce a word, ask the teacher.

PARTNER A

1. Listen and check:

   aid   _____

   I'd   _____

   add   _____

2. Pronounce:

   pet

   put

   <u>pat</u>

3. Listen and check:

   lift   _____

   left   _____

   laughed   _____

4. Pronounce:

   barn

   <u>born</u>

   burn

5. Listen and check:

   bruise   _____

   blaze   _____

   blues   _____

6. Pronounce:

   girt

   heart

   <u>hurt</u>

7. Listen and check:

   park   _____

   pork   _____

   perk   _____

8. Pronounce:

   sore

   <u>sure</u>

   sour

9. Listen and check:

ice	_____
eyes	_____
ace	_____

10. Pronounce:

called

cold

<u>sold</u>

11. Listen and check:

runs	_____
rungs	_____
wrens	_____

12. Pronounce:

<u>wetter</u>

waiter

water

13. Listen and check:

feels	_____
fills	_____
falls	_____

14. Pronounce:

cling

<u>clean</u>

clan

Demonstrations
(group activity)

A local TV station has asked your class to explain and demonstrate first aid procedures for a special program on first aid. In groups of 3 or 4, decide how you are going to present your demonstration:

○ cut on an arm, some bleeding
○ severe bleeding from cut on leg
○ small child swallows turpentine
○ a broken arm
○ an unconscious person
○ a nosebleed

In your demonstration, someone should introduce your topic, someone should be the injured person, one or two people should administer the first aid, and someone should give a review summary at the end. Use the following form to make your plans.

> **?** **Preliminary Planning Questionnaire**
>
> 1. What is your topic? _____
>
> 2. Who will introduce your topic, and how will they do it?
>
>   _____
>
>   _____
>
>   _____
>
> 3. Who will demonstrate the first aid, and how will they do it?
>
>   _____
>
>   _____
>
>   _____
>
> 4. Who will present the review at the end, and how will they do it?
>
>   _____
>
>   _____
>
>   _____
>
> 5. What "props" do you need to bring to class?
>
>   _____
>
>   _____
>
>   _____

Conversation
(pair activity)

Partner A will start the following conversation (question 1). Partner B must then decide which response (question 2, a or b) is appropriate. Partner A will then respond with the appropriate response (question 3, a or b) to Partner B and so on. The conversation will not make sense unless the right choices are made.

PARTNER A

1. Ouch! I just burned my arm as I was reaching inside the oven. What should I do?

3. a. I have a refrigerator but it doesn't work very well. I'm afraid it's not safe. The electrical wiring is bad.

   b. Yes, there is some in the freezer. Be careful not to cut yourself on the door. It has a sharp edge.

5. a. First you need to press against the cut with a clean paper towel. Hold your hand above your head until you can wash it, and then put on a Band-Aid. The Band-Aids are in the bathroom.

   b. Here, wrap it tightly in this old rag and keep it low down, beneath your heart. That way it won't bleed as much, and you won't even need a bandaid.

PARTNER B

2. a. You should be more careful. Do you have some butter we could put on it?

   b. Put it under cold water immediately. Do you have any ice?

4. a. Ouch! I see what you mean. Now I've cut my finger. What should I do?

   b. Sorry. I didn't mean to hurt your feelings. Do you want some soap?

6. a. All right. Here's some ice. Put it on your arm until I can come back to help you.

   b. O.K. Now you just sit down, lean forward and pinch your nose until I can help you with that burn.

8

911 Emergency Services

WORD LIST

Things

brakes
sidewalk
pay phone
emergency
receiver
dial tone
cross street
ambulance
electric shock
heart attack
assistance

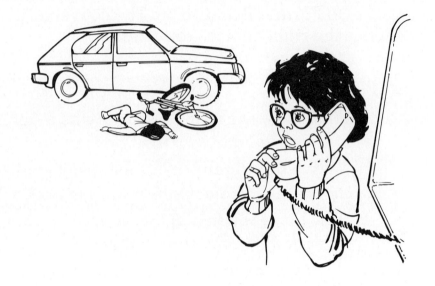

Actions

scare
slam
pounding
shaking
choking
drowning

Locations

next to

It's Saturday morning. Mark and Cathy are waiting at the library for their mother to pick them up. Cathy is outside sitting on a bench reading a book, but Mark is inside talking and laughing with some of his friends. Just then a car going too fast comes around the corner next to the library. The noise of the car scares Cathy. She looks up just as a boy on a bicycle goes out into the street. The driver slams on his brakes, but he hits the boy's bicycle and the boy falls off. Some people on the sidewalk come running. The boy isn't moving.

Cathy's heart is pounding. She's very scared, but suddenly she sees the pay phone next to the bench and she remembers what her mother told her to do in an emergency. She reaches up high and picks up the receiver. Her hand is shaking. She listens for the dial tone, then pushes the buttons 9–1–1. She doesn't need coins for an emergency call.

911: 911 Emergency.

Cathy: A car hit a boy on a bicycle.

911: What number are you calling from?

Cathy: 866-2315.

911: What's the address there?

Cathy: 3rd Avenue., in front of the library.

911: What's the cross street?

Cathy: B Street, I think.

911: What's your name?

Cathy: Cathy Santos.

911: We'll take care of it.

Mark comes running out of the library. He's saying, "What's the matter? What happened? Are you O.K.? Mom would kill me if you got hurt!"

Comprehension Check

Circle the correct answer:

1. Cathy is inside the library.

   a. true   b. false

2. What's Mark doing?

   a. He's reading a book.   b. He's laughing and talking with his friends.

   c. He's sitting on the bench outside the library.

3. What happened?

   a. A car hit a bicycle.   b. A bicycle hit a car.

   c. A car hit Cathy.

4. What does Cathy do after the accident?

  a. She goes to get Mark.   b. She calls an ambulance.

  c. She calls 911.

5. She doesn't need money for an emergency call.

  a. true   b. false

Cultural Note

  Call 911 for *any* serious health emergency such as bleeding, burns, broken bones, choking, drowning, electric shock, heart attack, or poisoning. Help should arrive in less than five minutes in most communities. Don't worry about what kind of assistance you need. The 911 operator will call an ambulance, a fire truck, or the police for you. Just answer all the questions the operator asks you, and let the operator finish the conversation.

Look at the picture and map below, then write the answers to the questions.

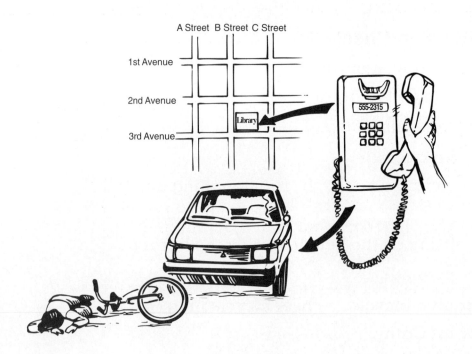

1. What number is Cathy calling? _____

2. Where is Cathy? _____

3. What's the cross street? _____

4. What number is she calling from? _____

5. What is Cathy using? _____

Practice answering these questions using your own information:

6. What number are you calling from? _____

7. What's the address? _____

8. What's the cross street? _____

9. What happened? (choose)

    a. A car hit someone.

    b. A man had a heart attack.

    c. Someone is choking.

    d. My son drank poison.

    e. My house is on fire.

    f. A woman is drowning.

10. What's your name? (first and last name) _____

11. What's your phone number? _____

Activity

Find your local emergency telephone number(s), write them down, and put them next to your telephone.

Multiple Choice

Circle the correct answer.

1. The part of a telephone you hold in your hand.

   receiver   dial tone

2. What is the sound a telephone receiver makes when you

   pick it up?   pay phone   dial tone

3. An accident that happens in the water:

   drowning   choking

4. What is another name for an accident?

ambulance   emergency

5. An accident when a piece of food stops your breathing:

choking   heart attack

6. Another name for "help":

assistance   shaking

7. An accident that happens when you touch something with an electrical current:

heart attack   electric shock

8. A truck or van that brings assistance in an emergency:

ambulance   sidewalk

Grammar 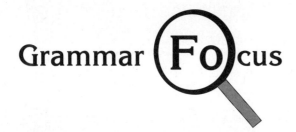 Focus

Use of "but"

We use the word "but" after a statement when we want to make another statement that seems opposite.

For example: She is tired, but she is going to work.

Choose a statement from the list to complete the sentences below:

For example: Cathy is outside the library, but _____.
Cathy is outside the library, but <u>Mark is inside</u>.

I can help   he couldn't stop
I'm learning   the nights are cool
she calls 911

1. Cathy is scared, but _____.

2. The days are hot, but _____.

3. The driver slammed on his brakes, but _____

_____.

4. School is difficult, but _____.

5. He knows there's a lot of work to do, but _____

_____.

What about you?

 ○ Do you have a 911 emergency services number where you
  live?

 ○ If you do not have a 911 number, do you know where to find
  emergency numbers in your telephone directory?

—— PRACTICE EXERCISES ——

Giving Information to 911
(pair activity)

Ask your partner for the information for your blank boxes. Use the conversation below. Write the information in your boxes. Partner B's chart is in Appendix A, page 224. *Do not look at your partner's page.*

PARTNER A

A: What is _____ 's _____?

B: His/Her _____ is _____.

Name	Phone No.	Problem	Address	Cross Street
Maria	313-9124		707 Elm St., Apt. 3B	
Juan		father having a heart attack	1691 W. 16th St.	
Samuel	847-2250			21st St.

Pair Interviews

Ask your partner the following questions and write the answers.

1. Have you ever been involved in an emergency, or do you know someone who has? What happened?
2. Did you ever have to call 911 for any reason? If yes, why?
3. What mistakes do you think people make when calling 911?
4. What is your favorite movie or TV program about an emergency situation?

Find Someone in the Class Who . . .

1. had to call 911 _____
2. needs to hold a practice fire drill at home _____
3. drives too fast _____
4. has been in an accident _____
5. knows CPR _____
6. knows the Heimlich maneuver _____
7. can ride a bicycle _____
8. has a library card _____
9. knows where to find emergency numbers in the phone book _____
10. watches "911" on TV every week _____

Role Play

Act out the following situations (in groups of 3 or 4). *Note:* In each group, one person must act as the 911 operator. That person must be sure to get all the necessary information. Supply your own information if it is not provided in the description.

1. At a child's birthday party at 119 Sanders Lane, one of the guests chokes on a piece of candy. The mother panics as the child turns blue, and the next-door neighbor must call 911.

2. A robber enters a store at the corner of Pine Ave. and 32nd St. and demands money from the store owner. When the owner refuses, the robber stabs him/her with a knife and runs away. The only customer in the store must call 911 as the seriously injured owner lies bleeding to death.

3. A babysitter suddenly smells smoke coming from one of the children's bedrooms. She/he quickly discovers that there is a fire in the baby's room. She/he grabs the baby and wakes the 7-year-old son, but as she/he calls 911 she/he realizes that she/he does not know the address, and the phone number is not written on the phone. She/he must get this information from the 7-year-old as she is talking to the 911 operator.

4. A man and a woman are driving down 8th Street in their car. Because they are having an argument, they do not see the bicycle rider who is trying to cross the street in front of them. The car hits the bicycle rider and breaks both of his/her legs. Someone must call 911 immediately.

5. A friend pulls a teenage surfer out of the water and onto the beach. The surfer is not breathing, and no one can hear a heartbeat. The surfer's friend speaks no English but knows the exact location of the beach. The friend must get an English-speaking tourist to talk to the 911 operator. The tourist does not know the exact location of the beach.

6. A customer at the Grandview Restaurant on Ocean Drive suddenly has a heart attack. While the waiter tries to make the person comfortable, a customer calls 911. (The waiter knows the exact address and the nearest Cross Street.)

7. A live electrical wire falls onto the stage of the Star Theater at 55th Street and Main, where a famous dancer is performing. The dancer falls unconscious from electrical shock. The stage manager runs out and begs someone from the audience to call 911. Since the electricity has been cut off, the audience person must dial in the dark and give the information.

8. An artist has a friend over for dinner. While they are talking and eating, the friend's child wanders off and drinks the artist's turpentine. The child begs for something to drink to make the pain go away. The child's parent is panic-stricken and also furious with the artist for leaving the turpentine out. The artist calls 911 and keeps calm with two people screaming at him/her.

Unit 2

COMMUNITY HEALTH SERVICES

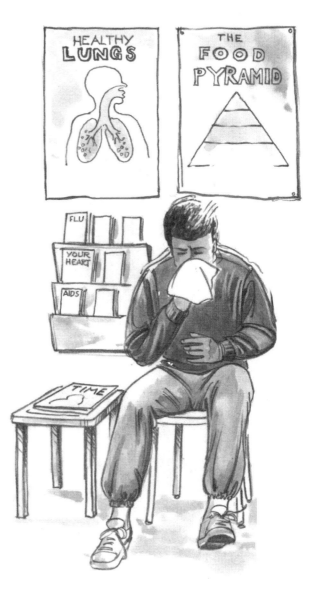

Visiting a Health Services Clinic

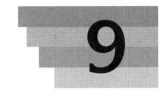

9

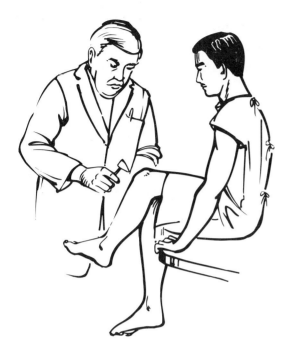

WORD LIST

Things
health services clinic
neighborhood
health history
paycheck stub
fee
income
sliding scale
allergy
surgery
hospitalization
blood pressure
pulse
abdomen
urine

patients
welfare
private hospital
immunization
tuberculosis

venereal disease
drug abuse
alcohol abuse
vaccination
treatment

The Santos family just moved to another city. That means new jobs for Tomas and Theresa, new schools for Mark and Cathy, new friends, a new neighborhood, a new health services clinic, and a new dentist. It's a difficult time for them with so many changes.

Today Tomas is going to a health services clinic for a physical examination. His new employer wants information on his physical health.

Tomas is upset. The cars in front of him are stopping all the time and he's supposed to be at the clinic 30 to 45 minutes before his appointment to fill out papers. He doesn't like being late. He also knows the doctor is going to tell him to stop smoking. "I've tried that before," he thinks.

At the clinic, the receptionist gives him a health information form to fill out about his health history. She also asks him for a paycheck stub to show his income and asks him how many people are in his family. Fees at a health services clinic are usually on a sliding scale so someone with a low income or many children may pay less than the regular fee.

The doctor asks Tomas more questions about his health history such as any drug allergies, surgeries, or hospitalizations. He takes Tomas's blood pressure and pulse. He looks in Tomas's eyes, mouth, nose, and ears. He feels his neck and abdomen. And last, Tomas gives a blood sample and a urine sample for testing.

"Your health's good," the doctor tells Tomas. "We'll call you if your samples show any problems. Your pulse is a little high, but if you stop smoking, I'm sure it'll go down."

Comprehension Check

Circle the correct answer.

1. What did the Santos family just do?

   a. go to a health services clinic   b. move to a new city

   c. go to a new dentist

2. Tomas knows the doctor will tell him to _____

   a. stop smoking   b. lose weight   c. exercise

3. What does the receptionist give Tomas?

   a. a paycheck stub   b. a health history   c. a health information

                                                          form

4. Everyone pays the same fee for a physical examination at a health services clinic.

   a. true   b. false

5. The doctor tells Tomas his _____ is high.

   a. pulse   b. blood pressure   c. weight

More Information

A health services clinic offers many services on a sliding fee scale, and usually there are no fees to patients on welfare. Services at a health services clinic are less expensive than at a private hospital. They may include immunization, eye exams, ear exams, dental clinic, physical examinations, family planning, well child clinic, tuberculosis testing and treatment, venereal disease testing and treatment, AIDS testing and treatment, drug abuse, alcohol abuse, vaccinations.

Call your local county health clinic for more information.

Word Groups

Cross out the word that does not belong.

1. allergy   hospitalization   drug abuse   alcohol abuse
2. abdomen   immunization   vaccination   treatment
3. pulse   urine   blood pressure   allergy
4. fee   patients   income   sliding scale
5. venereal disease   tuberculosis   welfare   surgery

Matching

Match the word with the meaning:

1. _____ when you go to the doctor your pulse and _____ are checked
2. _____ an area where families live
3. _____ drinking too much
4. _____ people the doctor takes care of
5. _____ what it costs to visit the doctor
6. _____ where you go for a physical exam
7. _____ a health information form is used to get the patient's _____
8. _____ the fee paid is based on how much your income is
9. _____ this paper will show how much money you earn
10. _____ one of the services you can get at a health services clinic

a. neighborhood
b. sliding scale
c. alcohol abuse
d. health history
e. blood pressure
f. immunization
g. paycheck stub
h. patients
i. health services clinic
j. fee

Grammar 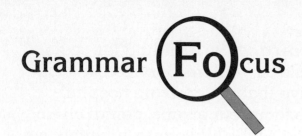cus

Contractions

Contractions can combine verbs and their subjects.

For example: you're—you are
he's—he is
we'll—we will

Fill in the blanks in the following sentences with contractions.

For example: (You are) _____ a good student.
<u>You're</u> a good student.

1. (It is) _____ raining.
2. Today (you are) _____ going to the clinic.
3. (It is) _____ a difficult time for them.
4. (They are) _____ stopping for dinner on the way home.
5. (I have) _____ tried that before.
6. (We are) _____ going to the movies tonight.
7. This afternoon (he is) _____ going to go for a physical examination.
8. (You are) _____ supposed to fill out these papers.

Activities

1. Find the address of your local county hospital.
2. Write down directions from your house or apartment to the county hospital.
3. Call the county hospital and ask any of these questions:
   a. Do you need insurance to get treatment?
   b. Do you have a sliding fee scale?
   c. Can I get treatment if I have no money?
   d. Can a person under 18 years old go for treatment without a parent?
   e. What are your hours?

Bingo

(group activity)

Make your own Bingo card (5 squares by 5 squares). Put one "Free" spot in the middle square. Then fill the other squares at random with the *past tenses* of some of the following verbs (if you don't know what they are, find out).

see	be	think	drive	forget	fall
make	try	catch	find	put	sit
do	begin	take	feel	buy	stand
go	give	come	shake	cut	
get	know	speak	leave	hold	
have	write	teach	say	dry	

		FREE		

The caller will say "Today I **see**; yesterday, I _____." If you have "saw" in one of your squares, put a marker on it. The first player to have one whole row of markers is the winner.

After you have played the game with the past tense, make a new card with the *past participles* of the verbs. For this game, the caller will say, "At present, I **see**; in the past I have _____." If you have "seen" in one of your squares, place a marker on it. Again, the object is to get a whole row of markers. Variations: markers in all four corners, in an "X" formation, or around all four edges.

Find Someone in the Class Who . . .

Copy the following chart. Then listen carefully as your teacher asks you questions. Then ask the same questions of your classmates until you find someone who has done what you are asking. Remember to change the first word (verb) to the past participle when you ask the question. Fill in the name of the person and the approximate time.

For example (for "go to a clinic"): "Have you ever **gone** to a clinic?"

Have You Ever . . .

What	Who	When
1. move to a new neighborhood		
2. make new friends		
3. go to a new school		
4. get a new job		
5. go to a health services clinic		
6. go to a dentist		
7. have a physical checkup		
8. have to wait a long time in a clinic		
9. be in a traffic jam		
10. arrive late for an appointment		
11. smoke cigarettes		
12. try to quit smoking cigarettes		
13. fill out a health form		
14. have surgery		
15. have an allergy to a drug		

Past Tense vs. Past Participle
(pair activity)

Study the following verb forms carefully. Then listen and choose the correct answer as your partner asks you questions. Only one of the choices is grammatically correct. Ask your partner questions and make sure that you both agree on which answer is correct.

Present	Past	Present/Perfect
move	moved	has/have moved
smoke	smoked	has/have smoked
make	made	has/have made
go	went	has/have gone
get	got	has/have gotten
have	had	has/have had
be	was/were	has/have been

PARTNER A

1. Listen and answer:
   a. Yes, I moved there last week.
   b. No. I hasn't moved there yet.
2. Ask: Have you ever gone to a hospital?
3. Listen and answer:
   a. No, she hasn't had one yet.
   b. Yes, she have had one last week.
4. Ask: Have they made any new friends?
5. Listen and answer:
   a. Yes, he got one yesterday.
   b. No, he haven't got one yet.
6. Has she ever smoked cigarettes?
7. Listen and answer:
   a. Yes, I been in one, but it wasn't too bad.
   b. Not today, but I have been in one before.

PARTNER B

1. Ask: Have you moved to your new apartment yet?
2. Listen and answer:
   a. No, I haven't went there yet.
   b. Yes, I went to one last week.
3. Ask: Has she had a physical checkup?
4. Listen and answer:
   a. Yes, they maked some this morning.
   b. No, they haven't made any yet.
5. Ask: Has he got a new job?
6. Listen and answer:
   a. No, she haven't ever smoked
   b. No, she hasn't ever smoked.
7. Ask: Were you in a traffic jam?

10 Visiting a Dentist

WORD LIST

Things
kids
waiting room
fluoride
floss
discomfort

Actions
prevent
shake hands

Descriptions
afraid
fearful
upset

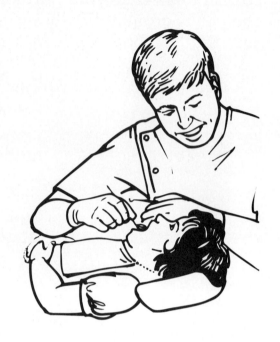

Cathy is leaving school a little early today. She likes school, especially reading, but today she doesn't mind missing a few minutes. She liked the kids at her other school better and her new teacher isn't as nice. This afternoon she's going to a new dentist, too. Everybody is new!

Her mother is picking her up at school since she hasn't found a new job yet.

"What's the dentist going to do?" Cathy is asking her mother.

"He's just going to look at your teeth. And he might take some pictures of them with a special camera."

"Will he have books for me in the waiting room like our old dentist?"

Dr. Oliver does have books and magazines for Cathy to look at while her mother talks to the receptionist and fills out a form about Cathy's health.

Dr. Oliver is coming into the waiting room to meet Cathy and her mother. He is smiling and shaking hands with both of them. Theresa stays in the waiting room while Cathy goes into

Dr. Oliver's office. Cathy is a little afraid, but Dr. Oliver explains that he wants to see only her so they can get to know each other.

When the dentist is finished taking X-rays, looking at Cathy's teeth, and cleaning them, he treats them with fluoride to prevent tooth decay. Then he gives Cathy a new toothbrush, and he lets her pick any color she wants.

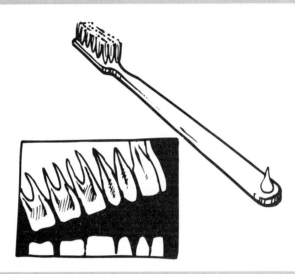

Afterwards he explains to Cathy and her mother the results of the X-rays and also how Cathy should brush and floss her teeth the right way. Theresa understands that Dr. Oliver wants to keep Cathy's teeth healthy more than he wants his money.

Comprehension Check

Circle the correct answer:

1. Why is Cathy leaving school early?

   a. because she's going to the dentist

   b. because she doesn't like school

   c. because her teacher isn't nice

2. Cathy likes her school.

   a. false   b. true

3. Is the dentist nice to her?

   a. Yes, he is.   b. No, he isn't.

4. What doesn't the dentist do?

    a. take X-rays   b. brush Cathy's teeth

    c. clean Cathy's teeth

5. Does Theresa trust Dr. Oliver?

    a. No, she doesn't.   b. Yes, she does.

More Information

Children and sometimes adults too are often afraid of going to the dentist. Usually they get this fear because they listen to someone talk about going to the dentist in a fearful way. They talk about pain or discomfort. Many times parents pass their fear on to their children without knowing it.

If you or your child has a fear of the dentist, tell your dentist. He can help you. Many people feel this way. Don't stay away because you're afraid. If your child is very upset when the dentist sees him, go home and try again another day.

Usually dental work causes no pain. And dentists almost never pull teeth anymore.

Fill in the Blank

Fill in the blanks with the correct words from the list below.

fearful	afraid	floss	kids
discomfort	upset	waiting room	prevent

    If you brush and (1) _____ your teeth correctly

every day, you can help (2) _____ tooth decay in

your own teeth. Your teeth will also give you less

(3) _____ and you don't have to be so

(4) _____ when you're sitting in the dentist's

(5) _____ _____. But some adults

and some (6) _____ are very much

(7) _____ of going to the dentist. Some people are

so (8) _____ they don't go to the dentist at all, but-

that can mean more problems.

Grammar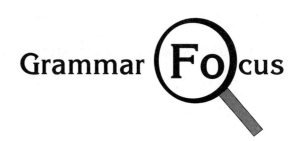

Possessive

The possessive is used to show ownership. Form the possessive of nouns by adding "'s" to the noun of ownership.

For example: Basilio's office is downtown. (Meaning: the office that belongs to Basilio)

Form the possessive of pronouns as follows:

I—my	she—her
you—your	we—our
he—his	they—their

For example: <u>Her</u> desk is in the corner. (Meaning: the desk that belongs to her)

Write the possessive form in each blank.

For example: the school that belongs to Cathy: <u>Cathy's school</u>

1. the office that belongs to the dentist _____

2. the mother that belongs to Cathy

3. the books and magazines that belong to Dr. Oliver

_____

4. the office that belongs to the receptionist_____

5. the dentist that belongs to him _____

6. the friends that belong to Mark _____

7. the teeth that belong to us_____

8. the jobs that belong to them _____

What about you?

○ How often do you go to the dentist?

○ Do you know how to take care of your teeth to keep them healthy?

○ Are you afraid of the dentist?

○ Are your children afraid of the dentist?

═══════ PRACTICE EXERCISES ═══════

Interview: What are You Most Afraid of?
(pair activity)

Look at the following problems associated with going to the dentist. Ask your partner to rank his/her fears from greatest (# 1) to least (# 6). Fill in the following information:

Fears:

having a toothache	getting a Novocain shot
dentist's drill	getting an X-ray
having a tooth pulled	getting the dentist's bill

MY PARTNER'S NAME:_____

MY PARTNER'S FEARS:

1. _____
2. _____
3. _____
4. _____
5. _____
6. _____

Now fill in the following information for the whole class:

NUMBER OF PEOPLE WHOSE GREATEST FEAR IS . . .

Having a toothache   _____

Dentist's drill   _____

Having a tooth pulled   _____

Getting a Novocain shot   _____

Getting an X-ray   _____

Getting the dentist's bill   _____

First Person, Third Person, and Questions

(pair activity)

Copy the following sentences and fill in the blanks with the correct verbs. Practice reading these sentences out loud to your partner.

For example: I brush my teeth every morning.
She <u>brushes</u> her teeth every morning.
<u>Does</u> she <u>brush</u> her teeth every morning?

1. I have dental insurance.

   He _____ dental insurance.

   _____ he _____ dental insurance?

2. I have three cavities.

   He _____ three cavities.

   How many cavities _____ he _____?

3. I have had X-rays often.

   He _____ _____ X-rays often.

   How often _____ he _____ X-rays?

4. I like my dentist because he's painless.

   He _____ his dentist because he's painless.

   Why _____ he _____ his dentist?

5. I am going to look at your teeth now.

   He _____ _____ to look at your teeth now.

   When _____ he _____ to look at your teeth?

6. I don't have any magazines in my waiting room.

   He _____ _____ any magazines in his waiting room.

   What _____ he _____ in his waiting room?

7. I go into the waiting room to meet new patients.

   He _____ into the waiting room to meet new patients.

   Where _____ he _____ to meet new patients?

Conversation: Formulating Questions
(pair activity)

Partner A will start the following conversation (question #1). Partner B must then decide which response (#2, a or b) is appropriate. Partner A will then respond with the appropriate response (#3, a or b) to Partner B, and so on. Pay close attention to the order of the words in the questions.

PARTNER A

1. Look! Cathy is leaving school early. Where *is she going*?

3. a. Because she hasn't found a job yet. What the dentist is going to do?

   b. Because she hasn't found a job yet. What is the dentist going to do?

5. a. I don't like X-rays. What time is her appointment?

   b. I don't like X-rays. What time her appointment is?

7. a. Because he always finds a new cavity. How you like having your teeth drilled?

   b. Because he always finds a new cavity. How do you like having your teeth drilled?

9. a. I guess I should. How you would tell him?

   b. I guess I should. How would you tell him?

PARTNER B

2. a. To my dentist. I recommended him. But why her mother is taking her?

   b. To my dentist. I recommended him. But why is her mother taking her?

4. a. He's going to take some X-rays. Why are you making that face?

   b. He's going to take some X-rays. Why you are making that face?

6. a. 1:30 p.m. Why don't you like X-rays?

   b. 1:30 p.m. Why you don't like X-rays?

8. a. I don't. Why you don't tell your dentist how you feel?

   b. I don't. Why don't you tell your dentist how you feel?

10. a. I'd say, "Doctor, I'm afraid of the drill. Can you please be very careful?"

    b. I'd say, "Doctor, I'm afraid of the drill. You can please be very careful?"

The Questioning Reporter
(pair activity)

A TV reporter is interviewing a person who is standing outside the dentist's office. The person has an appointment to see the dentist. Write down the dialogue between the reporter and the person who is about to see the dentist. Practice saying the dialogue, and then present your interview in front of the class.

REPORTER: Good afternoon, ladies and gentlemen. This is your ace reporter, _____(name)_____, coming to you *live* from outside the office of Dr. Dennis Bill. Standing next to me is one of his patients, _____(name)_____, and I'm going to ask him/her a few questions. Tell me what _____.

PATIENT: _____.

REPORTER: I see. When _____?

PATIENT: _____.

REPORTER: Where _____?

PATIENT: _____?

REPORTER: Why _____?

PATIENT: _____.

REPORTER How _____?

PATIENT: _____.

REPORTER: Thank you very much Mr./Ms. _____(name)_____. This is _____(name)_____ signing off for now. Back to you at the station, Ted.

(*Note:* If it suits your dialogue better, you may put the questions in different order. Just be sure to include "what," "when," "where," "why," and "how.")

11 Getting Glasses

WORD LIST

Things

glasses
road signs
stock numbers
optometrist
eye examination
advertisement
discount
lenses
frames
optician
style
contact lenses
vision

Actions

squint
lose

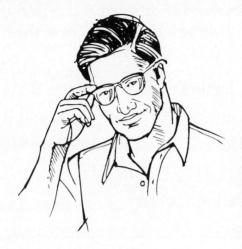
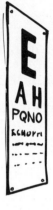
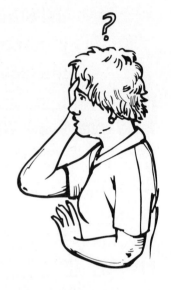

Tomas is having a little trouble reading the road signs on his way home from work. Also, in his new job as store manager he has to read a lot of stock numbers and he can't see the numbers very well. He knows he should see an optometrist for an eye examination, but he doesn't want to take time away from his new job. There is so much to do and so many new things to learn. Besides, he thinks he's too young to wear glasses!

One day he sees an advertisement in the newspaper for 10% off at the optometrist in a department store near his work. So Tomas makes an appointment because he is beginning to get headaches. He is happy to have an evening appointment so he doesn't have to miss work.

"I'm tired of squinting," Tomas tells the optometrist who is examining his eyes.

After the examination, the optometrist gives Tomas a prescription for lenses. Tomas can get the lenses made and choose the frames there, or he can take the prescription to an optician. But Tomas decides to buy them there because of the 10% discount, even though he can buy lenses and frames in many places. He is thinking mainly about cost because his wife isn't working yet. Still he has many frames and prices to choose from. He chooses carefully because he doesn't want to look old in his glasses.

Comprehension Check

Circle the correct answer.

1. What is Tomas having trouble with?

    a. doing his new job   b. reading the newspaper

    c. reading road signs

2. What does Tomas need?

    a. an eye examination   b. a new job   c. new things to learn

3. Tomas goes to an _____.

    a. optician   b. optometrist

4. The optometrist gives Tomas _____.

    a. lenses   b. frames   c. a prescription

5. When Tomas buys frames, which is more important to him?

    a. price   b. style

 # Cultural Note

Many Americans chose to wear contact lenses instead of glasses. Contact lenses are more trouble to put on than glasses, but many people like the fact that you can't see them. Maybe people feel, like Tomas, that glasses make them look older. And in America most people over 30 want to look *younger*, not older.

Contact lenses may also help keep your vision from getting worse. And they may improve vision more than glasses. But they are more difficult to take care of than glasses, and because they are so small, they are easy to lose.

Vocabulary Builder

Circle the correct word and write the word in the blank.

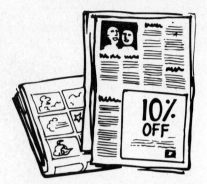

frames   stock numbers
advertisement

_____

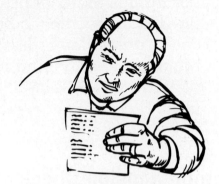

squint   lose
discount

_____

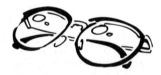

eye examination   glasses
vision

_____

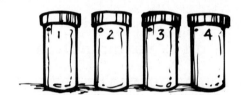

stock numbers   road signs
advertisement

_____

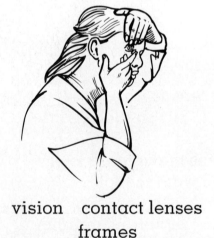

vision   contact lenses
frames

_____

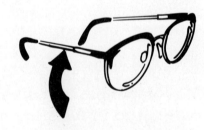

lenses   frames
contact lenses

_____

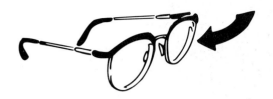

lose   squint
lenses

_____

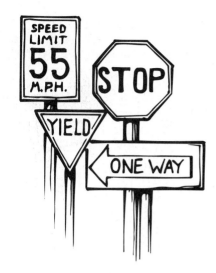

road signs   stock numbers
advertisement

_____

Fill in the Blank

Fill in the blanks with the correct words from the list.

optometrist	lenses
contact lenses	glasses
frames	optician
vision	squint
advertisements	eye examination

Armando can't see well. His (1) _____ is not
good. He thinks he needs (2) _____. He has to
(3) _____ to read the (4)_____ in the
newspaper. He goes to an (5) _____ to get an
(6) _____. Next he goes to an (7) _____
to get (8) _____ made and choose (9) _____
for them. He is getting glasses because (10) _____
are too hard to put in.

Crossword Puzzle

Fill in the words from the word list below.

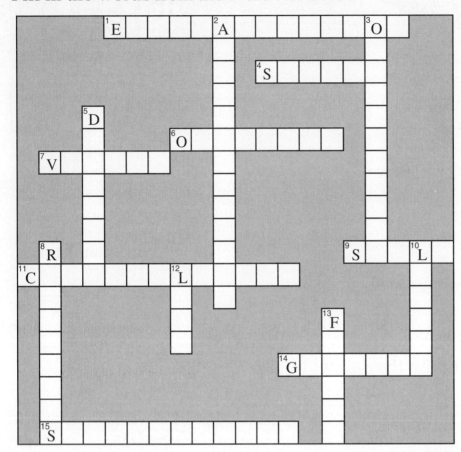

discount
vision
lose
eye examination
stock numbers
style
optometrist
contact lenses
optician
lenses
squint
frames
road signs
advertisement
glasses

ACROSS

1. when a doctor checks your eyes
4. when your eyes are almost closed
6. a person who makes glasses
7. your eyes give you _____
9. Tomas cares more about price than _____
11. these help you see better, like glasses
14. these will help Tomas see better
15. Tomas is having trouble reading the _____ at work

DOWN

2. Tomas saw an _____ in the newspaper.
3. a person who writes prescriptions for glasses
5. a lower price
8. you read traffic information on these
10. the frames hold the _____ in front of your eyes
12. contact lenses are small and easy to _____
13. these hold the lenses in a pair of glasses

Grammar 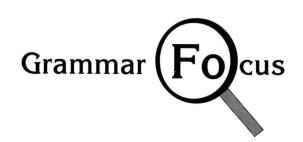cus

Present vs. Present Continuous

The present tense is used to express an action which goes on regularly or in general. The present continuous is used to describe an action that is going on right now.

For example: Present Tense: Tomas thinks he's too young to wear glasses. (Tomas thinks this in general.)

(*Note:* For regular verbs in the third-person singular present tense, add an "s" at the end of the verb. For regular verbs which end in "ch," "sh," "j," "s," "x," and "z," add "es.")

Present Continuous: Tomas is telling the optometrist he's tired of squinting. (Tomas is telling the optometrist right now.)

(*Note:* Form the present continuous by using the present tense form of the verb "to be" and adding "ing" to the base form of the main verb.)

Change the following present-tense sentences to the present continuous.

For example: Juan <u>walks</u> to work everyday. (present)
Juan <u>is</u> <u>walking</u> to work. (present continuous)

1. Tomas squints at work.

_____.

2. Tomas gets headaches reading stock numbers.

_____.

3. Tomas chooses his frames carefully.

_____.

4. He buys at a discount.

_____.

5. The optometrist gives Tomas a prescription for lenses.

_____.

What about you?

- ○ Have you ever had an eye examination?
- ○ Do you wear glasses or contact lenses? If so, did you go to an optician?
- ○ Do you think glasses look bad?
- ○ Do you think contact lenses are worth the extra trouble?

══════ PRACTICE EXERCISES ══════

Interview

(pair activity)

Ask your partner the following questions, and mark his/her responses in the appropriate box. Be sure to phrase your question correctly.

Examples:

Ask your partner . . .

1. if he/she is having trouble reading small print
   (You would say: *"Are you having trouble reading small print?"*)

2. if he/she sometimes has trouble with homework
   (You would say: *"Do you sometimes have trouble with homework?"*)

Ask your partner . . .	Yes	No
1. if he/she is having trouble reading the blackboard		
2. if he/she sometimes has trouble reading road signs		
3. if he/she has to read a lot on the job		
4. if he/she is thinking of seeing an optometrist		
5. if he/she thinks he/she is too young to wear glasses		
6. if he/she lives near his/her place of work		

	Yes	No
7. if he/she is getting a lot of headaches these days		
8. if he/she is enjoying this class		
9. if he/she knows anyone who wears contact lenses		
10. if he/she is squinting right now		
11. if he/she thinks glasses look bad		
12. if he/she is feeling good right now		

Now change partners and ask your new partner about his/her previous partner. Use the same chart.

Examples: 1. Is he/she having trouble reading small print?
2. Does he/she sometimes have trouble with homework?

Eye Chart
(pair activity)

This is a sample of an eye chart:

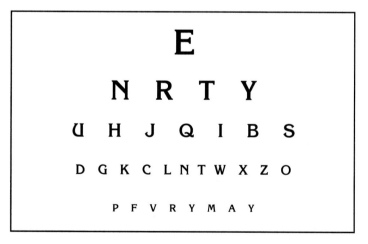

Make up your own eye chart and test your partner's vision. Be sure to include all the letters of the alphabet. Make the top letters very large. The bottom line should be very small. The chart should be far enough away so that the bottom line is difficult if not impossible to read. Your partner should cover one eye while reading off the letters. Then cover the other eye and repeat the process. Note how many errors are made.

Role Play

Act out the following situations (in groups of 3, 4, or 5). Be sure that everyone has something to say.

1. A family of four is riding in a car and looking for Elm Street. The driver is having trouble reading the signs, so he/she keeps missing Elm Street. The other people in the car try to show the driver where Elm Street is. Someone in the family has to convince the driver to get glasses so this won't happen again.

2. A parent is at the optometrist's with two children. The optometrist checks the eyesight of the children. One child can see perfectly but the other one needs glasses. The one who needs glasses does not want to wear glasses but says contact lenses would be O.K. The parent thinks that contacts are too expensive. The child with good vision makes fun of the child who needs glasses. How is the parent going to handle this problem?

3. A teacher is "dictating" sentences for students to write. The students are trying to write the sentences, but the teacher cannot see very well and keeps reading the lines differently. (First the teacher says, "To get hired for a job, you must be on time," and then "To get fired from a job, you must be in line." Next the teacher says, "Eye contact is very important," then "My contract is very important.") The students are very confused; they don't know what they are supposed to write. The students need to find a polite way to tell the teacher to get a new prescription for glasses.

4. Three people are playing basketball. A referee is with them. Player X suddenly loses a contact lens. He must find it on the floor before another player steps on it. The other players want to help but they don't know what a contact lens looks like, so Player X must describe it and tell them how to look for it without scratching it or breaking it. Meanwhile, the referee wants them to hurry up so the game can continue.

5. A teacher is over 45 years old and is having trouble reading small print or anything that is too close. Students keep putting papers in front of the teacher's face to read and the teacher must push the papers away in order to read them.

The teacher wonders if reading glasses might be a good idea, or maybe a magnifying glass. One problem, however, is that the teacher loses things all the time and she might lose the reading glasses or magnifying glass. The students suggest solutions.

6. An optician has three customers. One is a movie star who wants diamond-studded prescription sunglasses and is very anxious to find frames that will project a glamorous image. The second customer is a teenager who wants contact lenses that will change the color of his/her eyes. The third customer is a bank robber in the middle of a getaway. He/she needs a disguise—fast!

12 Visiting an Emergency Room

WORD LIST

Things

emergency room
medical insurance
form
examination room
tetanus shot
needle
stitches
pain
knife
nail

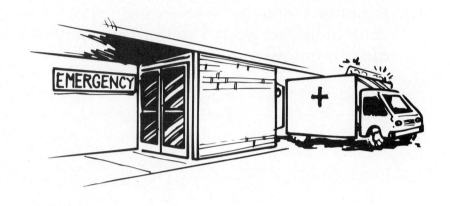

Actions

bother
inject
confuse

Descriptions

bloody
numb

metal
positively

It's Wednesday afternoon. Theresa is at home because she hasn't found a new job yet. She hears a knock on the door and opens it. Her new neighbor, Ana, is there with a bloody towel around her right hand.

"I'm sorry to bother you," she says, "but I cut my hand and the bleeding won't stop. Can you take me to the hospital? My English is no good."

"Of course. You can ask me for help any time. Where's the nearest hospital? I'm new here."

"I don't know. I can't read a map. But I need to go to the county hospital because I have no medical insurance."

"I know where that is," says Theresa. "You need to wrap the towel tight and put your hand up high. Everything's going to be fine." Ana looks a little scared.

At the emergency room, the receptionist says to Ana, "You need to fill out some forms." Ana doesn't understand why she has to fill out forms before she sees the doctor. She's getting upset. "My hand," she says, ". . . I can't write."

But Theresa helps her with the forms. "They need to know something about your medical history before they do anything," says Theresa.

Because Ana is bleeding, she doesn't have to wait as long as some of the other people in the emergency room.

In the examination room, the nurse asks Ana how she cut herself while he cleans the wound. He also asks if she has had a tetanus shot in the last ten years. Then he tells her the doctor will come soon.

The doctor examines Ana's hand and injects some medicine near the cut to numb it. Ana is scared of needles, but now she's also confused. The nurse is a man and the doctor is a woman!

When Ana's hand is numb, the doctor stitches the cut closed and puts a clean bandage on it. Just to be safe, she also gives Ana a tetanus shot.

Finally, the doctor gives Ana a prescription for some pain medicine. "Come back in a week and I'll take the stitches out," she tells Ana with a smile. "Everything's going to be fine."

Comprehension Check

Circle the correct answer.

1. What does Ana want?

   a. She wants a new job.   b. She wants to go to the emergency room.

   c. She wants to knock on Theresa's door.

2. Theresa is glad to help Ana.

   a. true   b. false

3. Why does Ana want to go to a county hospital?

   a. She has no medical insurance.   b. It's the nearest hospital.

   c. It costs more, but it's worth it..

4. Theresa tells Ana to _____.

   a. wrap the towel tight and put her hand up   b. take the towel off her hand

   c. relax her hand

5. The nurse asks Ana _____.

   a. to fill out forms   b. why she's upset

   c. when she last had a tetanus shot

6. What is Ana scared of?

   a. needles   b. pain medicine   c. stitches

7. What doesn't the doctor give Ana?

   a. a prescription   b. aspirin   c. a tetanus shot

More Information

An emergency room is for emergencies only. You don't need an appointment, but you should be ready to give your medical history when you go in. Don't go to an emergency room if you can wait for an appointment.

A county hospital will accept patients without medical insurance, but you must show that you cannot pay. Also, you may have to wait a long time in a county hospital, even in the emergency room.

You need a tetanus shot when something metal, like a knife or a nail, breaks your skin. But you only need a tetanus shot every ten years.

If you take someone to an emergency room, remember he/she usually feels scared. You can help by talking positively to him/her.

Activity

Write the name, address, and telephone number of the county hospital in your city.

_____

_____

_____

_____

Multiple Choice

Circle the correct answer.

1. A place you go for fast medical care without an appointment:

   examination room   emergency room

2. What do you need when you scratch yourself on metal?

   tetanus shot   needle

3. What do you need when a cut bleeds a lot?

   stitches   pain

4. A plan that pays some or all of your medical costs:

   medical insurance   form

5. A doctor gives a tetanus shot with a _____.

   nail   needle

6. What is a word that means "to put medicine in with a needle"?

   bother   inject

7. If you can't feel anything you feel _____.

   numb   bloody

8. "Everything's going to be fine" is an example of speaking

   _____.

   positively   negatively

9. If you don't understand you are _____.

   metal   confused

10. What is a piece of paper where you write information?

    a form   a knife

Grammar 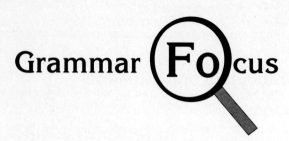cus

Use of "need to"

Use the expression "need to" when you want to express necessity.

For example: I need to go to a county hospital. (Meaning: it is necessary that I go)

Write five sentences about yourself using the expression "need to" and the phrases below.

For example: I need to <u>make</u> more money.

get a new job   go to the dentist   take a shower   fill out this form
go to the doctor   get some sleep   learn more   get to work on
                                                              English   time

1. I _____.

2. I _____.

3. I _____.

4. I _____.

5. I _____.

6. What do you need to do right now?

_____.

Fill in the following sample health information form.

Sample Health Information Form

_____

LAST NAME   FIRST NAME   MIDDLE INITIAL

_____

ADDRESS: NUMBER   STREET   CITY   STATE   ZIP CODE

_____   _____

DAY TELEPHONE   EVENING TELEPHONE

_____   _____ SEX: F____ M ____

SOCIAL SECURITY   BIRTHDATE
   NUMBER

In Case of Emergency, Call _____
                              NAME

_____

RELATIONSHIP   WORK PHONE   HOME PHONE

_____

NAME OF MEDICAL INSURANCE AND MEMBER NUMBER

Do you take any medications regularly? _____

Please list : _____

Do you have any allergies to food or medication? _____

Please list : _____

Why do you want to see a doctor?

_____

_____   _____

PATIENT SIGNATURE   DATE

What about you?

- ○ When do you go to an emergency room instead of calling 911?
- ○ Have you been in an emergency room? What was the emergency?
- ○ Do you know where the county hospital is in your city?
- ○ Do you have health insurance?

━━━━ PRACTICE EXERCISES ━━━━

Pronunciation Exercise
(pair activity)

Copy the following lists of words Partner A's are listed here. Partner B's are in Appendix A, pages 225-226. Where it says "Listen and check" put a check mark by the word your partner pronounces. Where it says "Pronounce" say only the word that is underlined, and your partner will put a check mark by that word. *Do not look at your partner's page.* When you are finished, correct your answers. If you don't know how to pronounce a word, ask the teacher.

PARTNER A

1. Listen and check:

bud   _____

blood   _____

brood   _____

2. Pronounce:

from

forum

<u>form</u>

3. Listen and check:

shock   _____

shake   _____

shook   _____

4. Pronounce:

<u>heart</u>

heard

hard

5. Listen and check:

scarred   _____

scored   _____

scared   _____

6. Pronounce:

shaking

chafing

<u>choking</u>

7. Listen and check:

droning _____

drowning _____

draining _____

8. Pronounce:

far

fair

<u>fear</u>

9. Listen and check:

pine _____

pain _____

pan _____

10. Pronounce:

<u>patients</u>

patents

passions

11. Listen and check:

fission _____

fashion _____

vision _____

12. Pronounce:

steal

stale

<u>style</u>

13. Listen and check:

rose _____

lose _____

loose _____

14. Pronounce:

loom

rum

<u>room</u>

Emergency!
(pair activity)

Ask your partner for the information for your blank boxes. Partner B's chart is in Appendix A, page 226. Use the conversation below. Write the information in your boxes.

PARTNER A

A: What did _____ do?

B: He/she has _____.

A: Where did he/she _____?

B: He/she _____ in _____

Name	What he/she did	Where
Jack Tripper	fell and he couldn't get up	
Mary Wanna		in an alley
Dee Livery	had a baby	
Kent Cutwright		in the hospital cafeteria

After you have found out all the necessary information from your partner, write out the following sentences by filling in the blanks correctly.

1. Jack Tripper has _____

   Where did he _____?

2. Mary Wanna has _____

   Where did she _____?

3. Dee Livery has _____

   Where did she _____?

4. Kent Cutwright has _____

   Where did he _____?

Dice Game
(group activity)

Taking turns, roll a die and move the number of spaces shown. If you land on an empty square, stay there and wait for your next turn. If you land on a square with a sentence, say whether it is correct or incorrect. If it is incorrect, correct it. If you are right, move ahead two squares. If you are incorrect, move back two squares.

FINISH 50	You need an appointment for the emergency room 49	You need a tetanus shot every 20 years. 48	47	Always hold a bleeding cut **below** your heart. 46
41	An optician is a person who makes glasses. 42	43	The word "pain" rhymes with "sign." 44	45
To "squint" means to open eyes very wide. 40	39	A "discount" is an error in counting. 38	37	Contact lenses are larger than glasses. 36
31	All people are afraid of going to the dentist. 32	33	34	An optician gives prescriptions for glasses. 35
30	29	"Sliding fee scale" means the same fees for everyone. 28	27	Fluoride prevents tooth decay. 26
You need insurance at a county hospital. 21	22	23	Today I **do**; yesterday I **done**. 24	25
20	You can find emergency numbers in the phone book. 19	18	Today I **see**; yesterday I **seen**. 17	16
You don't need money to call 911. 11	12	It's O.K. to make a crank call to 911. 13	14	A cross street is the same as a driveway. 15
10	Always give milk to a poison victim. 9	"Rum rhymes with"room." 8	7	Give an unconscious person lots of water. 6
START	Wash a serious burn with soap and very hot water. 1	Put ice on a bad bruise. 2	3	For serious bleeding, press on wound with a dirty cloth. 5

Unit 3

CHILDREN'S AND ADOLESCENTS' HEALTH

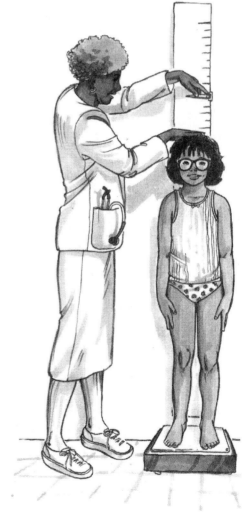

Vaccinations

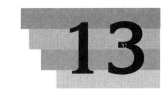

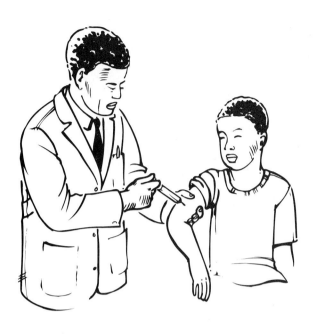

Things
members
garage
pneumonia
respiratory problems
record
service
immigration official
immunization
appetite

Actions
scratch
cut
require

Descriptions
necessary
slight

Because Ana got her tetanus shot in the emergency room, Theresa starts thinking about her family's vaccinations. Do all the members of the family have the vaccinations they need?

Theresa remembers that she had a tetanus shot about three years ago when she scratched her leg on a nail in the garage. But what about Tomas? He's always scratching or cutting himself when he works around the house and on the car. And what about vaccinations for pneumonia and the flu?

When she calls the Public Health Department they tell her that pneumonia and flu vaccinations (except for Hib meningitis) are only necessary for people over age 60 or people with respiratory problems. But they tell her where Tomas can get a tetanus shot if he needs one.

For each of the children, Theresa has a "vaccination record card." Mark and Cathy have both gotten all of the vaccinations they need. These are the recommended vaccinations:

Approximate Age	Vaccine
2 months	* DPT, oral polio, and ** Hib meningitis
4 months	DPT, oral polio, and Hib meinigitis
6 months	DPT, oral polio, and Hib meningitis
15 months	***MMR
18 months	DPT, MMR, and Hib meningitis
4 to 6 years	DPT, MMR, and oral polio
10 to 12 years	rubella (Only for females in special cases. See a doctor for more information.)
Every 10 years	DT
Every 7 years	**** Hepatitis B

* DPT = diphtheria, pertussis, tetanus

** Hib meningitis = Haemophilus influenza type b causing meningitis

*** MMR = measles, mumps, rubella

**** some children will also receive 3 Hepatitis B vaccines in their first year of life

Theresa is looking at the cards when Cathy comes home from school. She wants to read hers.

When Mark comes home, he thinks his mother worries too much about everybody's health. "Why worry? We all feel fine," he says.

Comprehension Check

Circle the correct answer.

1. Three years ago Theresa had a _____.

   a. tetanus shot   b. nail   c. garage

2. Do Theresa and Tomas need pneumonia and flu vaccinations?

a. yes   b. no

3. Mark and Cathy need pneumonia and flu vaccinations.

a. true   b. false

4. How many times did Mark and Cathy each go for vaccinations before they were two years old?

a. 2   b. 8   c. 5

5. Which vaccinations do Mark and Cathy need after age 12?

a. oral polio   b. measles, mumps, and rubella

c. tetanus, diphtheria, and Hepatitis B

6. Which vaccinations do people need only after age 60?

a. DPT and rubella   b. pneumonia and flu

c. oral polio and Hib meningitis

Cultural Note

All students who enter school in the United States must have all the required vaccinations before they can enter school. The Public Health Department will give any needed vaccinations. Sometimes this service is free.

For people coming from other countries, immigration officials will ask for their immunization record of vaccinations. The U.S. and many other countries even require vaccinations before you go to another country.

The required vaccinations in the U.S. for all school children are: polio, diphtheria, pertussis, tetanus, measles, mumps, rubella, and haemophilus influenza type b.

People over age 60 should have a pneumonia vaccination once, and a flu vaccination every fall.

Sometimes children and adults will get a little sick after a vaccination. They may have a slight fever, swelling near the vaccination, or loss of appetite. If the effects are worse, a doctor should be called.

Word Groups

Cross out the word that does *not* belong.

For example: red   blue   ~~color~~   green

1. decrease   official   require   cut
2. immigration   vaccination   immunization   record
3. appetite   polio   rubella   measles
4. pneumonia   diphtheria   problems   mumps
5. nail   cut   decrease   require

Multiple Choice

Circle the correct answer.

1. What are the people in a family called?

   problems   members

2. "A little bit" means

   slight   necessary

3. What does a vaccination sometimes cause?

   swelling   appetite

4. Which of these is a respiratory disease?

   vaccination   pneumonia

5. "Required" means:

   necessary   service

6. What can a nail do?

   decrease   scratch

7. What can prevent flu and pneumonia?

   a vaccination   an official

8. The Public Health Department gives needed vaccinations. What is this an example of?

   service   vaccination

Fill in the Blank

Fill in the blanks with the correct words from the list below.

flu	swelling
vaccination	respiratory
nail	immigration
required	record
immunization	scratched

1. A _____ will keep you from getting a disease.

2. An _____ record shows the vaccinations you have.

3. Theresa _____ her leg on a _____.

4. Sometimes when you get a vaccination there is _____ near the vaccination.

5. If someone has trouble breathing, he/she has _____ problems.

6. Theresa and Tomas do not need a _____ vaccination.

7. Mark's and Cathy's vaccination _____ cards show that they got the _____ vaccinations.

8. An _____ official will ask for your immunization record.

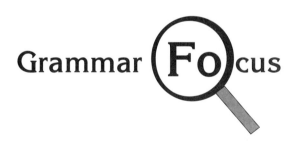

Grammar Focus

Use of "What about?"

The question "What about . . .?" is used to ask about the inclusion of someone or something.

For example: Abdel and Phuoc are going to the movies.
What about Lee? (Meaning: Is Lee going too?)

or

Theresa had a tetanus shot three years ago.
But what about Tomas? (Meaning: Did Tomas have one too?)

Write questions using the expression "what about" in the spaces below.

For example: Carlos is going shopping. Ask if Aida is going too.
<u>What</u> <u>about</u> <u>Aida</u>?

1. The baby has her oral polio vaccination. Ask if she has her DPT.

   _____.

2. Theresa worries about Tomas's health. Ask if she worries about Mark's and Cathy's health too.

   _____.

3. Food is expensive. Ask if rent is also expensive.

   _____.

4. Pilar works 60 hours a week. Ask about Kim.

   _____.

5. Theresa is looking at Cathy's vaccination record card. Ask if she is looking at Mark's too.

   _____.

What about you?
- ○ What vaccinations are required in your country?
- ○ What vaccinations do you have?
- ○ If you have children, what vaccinations do they have?

PRACTICE EXERCISES

Interview
(pair activity)

Ask your partner the following questions and write down their answers. You don't have to write every word they say—try to keep your sentences short and to the point. Be prepared to report your findings to the class.

1. Have you ever had a tetanus shot? If yes, why did you have it?

2. Are you afraid of getting a shot? How afraid? (not at all? a lot? a little bit?)

3. When was the last time you got a shot?

4. Do you have a vaccination record card?

5. Do you know someone who has tuberculosis?

6. Do you know someone who has had a flu shot? If yes, did it help?

7. What vaccinations are required in your native country?

8. What childhood diseases are the most common in your native country?

9. What childhood diseases have you had? (Examples: chicken pox, rubella, measles, mumps, whooping cough, pneumonia, flu, etc.)

10. Did you ever get sick after having a vaccination? If yes, what happened?

Conversation
(pair activity)

Study the information about vaccinations carefully and then figure out the correct answers to the following questions. You and your partner will take turns presenting the problem and choosing the correct solution from answers a, b, and c.

PARTNER A

1. (Read): Anita has stepped on a nail. The nail broke the skin.
2. (Answer): a. Before winter starts, she should probably have pneumonia and flu vaccinations.
    b. Before winter starts, she should probably have a tetanus shot.
    c. Before winter starts, she should probably have a DPT shot.
3. (Read): Baby Snookums is almost two months old. His mother is taking him to a clinic for a checkup.
4. (Answer): a. She will need to show proof that she has had DPT, MMR, and flu vaccinations.
    b. She will need to show proof that she has had pneumonia, flu, and MMR vaccinations.
    c. She will need to show proof that she has had DPT, MMR, and polio vaccinations.

PARTNER B

1. (Answer): a. She may need to have a DPT shot.
    b. She may need an oral polio vaccination.
    c. She may need a tetanus shot.
2. (Read): Grandma is 68 years old. During the winter she catches one cold after another.
3. (Answer): a. He will probably get a tetanus shot, if he has not already had one.
    b. He will probably get a DPT shot and oral polio vaccination.
    c. He will probably get a measles, mumps, and rubella vaccination.
4. (Read): Thirteen-year-old Sonia has just moved to the United States from Mexico. She will be entering an American school this fall.

Choral Reading: Song
(group activity)

The following should be sung to the tune of "She'll Be Comin' Round the Mountain." Half the class can sing the "Patient's Lament" and the other half the "Nurse's Reply." Try to pick up the rhythm of the words. This will help you pronounce better as well as remember the medical information.

Patient:
If you're comin' round with needles, go away!
If you're comin' round with needles, go away!
Though I need the vaccination
I give you this supplication
If you're comin' round with needles, go away!

Nurse:
Yes, I'm comin' round with needles, don't lament
So relax and just be glad we can prevent
Lots of awful old diseases
Like *rubella, mumps, and measles,*
 It will only hurt a little, don't lament.

Patient:
I have heard of those diseases, and it's true
That I ought to feel glad and not be rude
But that needle is so long and
I am anything but strong, so
I'll be going out the door now. Later, Dude!

 Nurse:
Let me tell you the diseases you might get
If you don't get vaccinated, don't forget:
You could come down with *diphtheria*
Now there's no need for hysteria
Just roll up your sleeve and you'll be in my debt.

Patient:
I know some of those diseases, and they're bad
Polio would make me very, very sad
Whooping cough is called pertussis,
And I see what all this fuss is
OK, do it, but be quick and I'll be glad.

Nurse:
Now I see you are a patient with good sense
You can look at life with much more confidence
With this shot which prevents *tetanus*
We'll be sure it won't be gettin' us
And against disease we do have some defense.

Continuous Line Drill

Your teacher will tell half the class to write the following on a piece of paper:

Example: Today he _____.
Yesterday he _____.
He has _____.

Next the teacher will tell those students to put one of the following verbs at the top of the paper (the teacher will assign each verb to a different student):

do	have	come
be	tell	think
get	worry	give
say	go	forget
feel	cut	know

Those students will then form an outside circle. The other half of the class will form an inside circle. When the teacher says, "Start," the people on the inside will move from one outside person to the next. They must look at the verb, then read each sentence, filling in and spelling the verb correctly before moving on. When everyone has gone around twice, the outside circle changes places with the inside circle, and the process is repeated.

For example: Verb: eat
The person on the inside will say:
Today he <u>eats</u>. "e - a - t - s"
Yesterday he <u>ate</u>. "a - t - e"
He has <u>eaten</u>. "e - a - t - e - n"

Be sure each person both reads the sentence correctly and spells the verb correctly.

School Physical

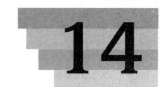
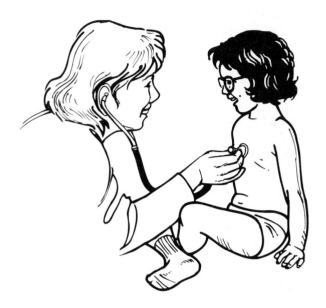

WORD LIST

Things
fruit
cookies
snack
stethoscope
urine
district
responsibility
guardian
result
waiver

Actions
try out
notice
protect
request

Descriptions
impatient
well developed
hearing

Because Mark and Cathy changed schools when they moved to another city, they have to get physical examinations. Mark also needs a physical because he is trying out for the basketball team. He doesn't understand why he needs an exam when he feels just fine. "But the *doctor* needs to know you're fine," Cathy is explaining to him.

During each of their exams, the doctor asks a lot of questions about their habits and their diets. Cathy thinks carefully about each question, but Mark is impatient. He thinks the doctor asks too many questions. But both Mark and Cathy are well-developed and of average weight and height, so the doctor isn't too worried. He does suggest fruit instead of cookies for snacks.

Next the doctor checks blood pressure, pulse, and respiration. He listens to the chest, front and back, with a stethoscope. He feels the abdomen and asks if anything hurts.

When the doctor is finished, Mark and Cathy each have to give a blood and a urine sample for tests. And they are given tuberculosis (TB) skin tests which have to be read in two days.

A nurse gives them each a hearing test and an eye test. Mark needs glasses like his father, but decides he wants contacts, ones that will make his eyes look really brown so the girls will notice him.

Comprehension Check

Circle the correct answer.

1. Why do Mark and Cathy need physical examinations?

   a. because they changed schools   b. because they didn't get their vaccinations

   c. because they don't feel well

2. What doesn't the doctor ask them about?

   a. their diets   b. their habits   c. their teeth

3. The doctor suggests _____ for snacks.

   a. cookies   b. fruit   c. peanut butter

4. What does the doctor use a stethoscope for?

   a. to check height   b. to take the temperature

   c. to listen to the chest

5. What samples do Cathy and Mark have to give?

   a. blood   b. urine   c. both a and b

6. After how many days are their tuberculosis skin tests read?

   a. 2   b. 5   c. 7

Cultural Note

To protect the health of all children, most states require a physical examination at the time a child enters school. If a student changes school districts he/she is usually required to get another exam.

A physical examination is the responsibility of the parent or guardian of the child. It is *not* the responsibility of the school. It is also the responsibility of the child's parent or guardian to give the results of the test to the school. If a parent does not want the child to have a physical, a waiver can be requested.

A physical, which may include a test for drugs, is usually required for participation in school sports programs as well.

Even if a child doesn't change schools, for protection he/she should have a physical according to the following schedule: age 4–5, age 6–8, age 9–12, age 13–16, age 17–20.

Call your local health services clinic or your doctor to make an appointment.

Matching

Match the word with the meaning.

1. _____ how tall you are
2. _____ food you eat between meals
3. _____ something you have to do
4. _____ the doctor listens to your chest with a _____
5. _____ what you eat
6. _____ after a test, you get the _____
7. _____ an adult (not a parent) who is responsible for a child
8. _____ to ask for
9. _____ a release
10. _____ an orange is a _____

a. fruit
b. responsibility
c. height
d. stethoscope
e. diet
f. waiver
g. request
h. guardian
i. snack
j. result

Grammar 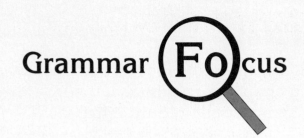cus

Use of "each" and "both"

Use "each" to talk about one item at a time.

For example: Cathy thinks carefully about <u>each</u> question. (Meaning: she thinks about the questions one at a time)

Use "both" to talk about two items together.

For example: Mark and Cathy <u>both</u> have to get physical examinations. (Meaning: the two of them)

Fill in the blanks with "each" or "both."

1. The doctor suggests we eat _____ fruits and vegetables.
2. _____ student in the class must take the test.
3. _____ Jorge and Juan were late for work.
4. Chu studies _____ lesson carefully.
5. Chu studies _____ lessons carefully.
6. _____ Mark and Cathy are of average height.
7. Let's take _____ children to the park.
8. _____ of the dogs had its own bed.

What about you?

○ Have you ever had a physical examination? If so, how long ago?

○ If you have children, have they had a physical examination?

PRACTICE EXERCISES

Let's Play Charades
(practice in asking questions)

The following activities will be written out on separate pieces of paper. The class will be divided into two teams. Two people at a time (from one team) will come up and act out the activity written on the piece of paper which the teacher will hand out. In order to win a point, someone on the actors' team must identify the activity *and* phrase the question correctly.

For example: "Are you reading an eye chart?"

filling out a questionnaire	checking his/her pulse
taking his/her temperature	checking his/her reflexes
listening to his/her heartbeat	checking his/her eyes
measuring his/her height	checking his/her throat
taking a blood sample	weighing him/her
giving a hearing test	giving a TB skin test
paying the bill	putting on contact lenses

Find Someone in the Class Who . . .

1. has had a physical examination in the last 12 months _____
2. has had his/her eyes tested for new glasses in the last 12 months _____
3. has had a hearing test in the last 12 months _____
4. is 5'4" tall _____
5. is happy with his/her weight _____
6. likes to eat fruit for snacks _____

7. hates to fill out questionnaires _____

8. has had to change schools 3 or more times _____

9. knows what a stethoscope is
   (and can tell you) _____

10. would like to have contact lenses _____

11. gets impatient while waiting to
    see the doctor _____

12. has tried out for a sports team _____

13. has sore feet _____

14. thinks you ask too many questions _____

15. wishes he/she could be taller _____

16. wishes he/she could be shorter _____

17. has never had a TB skin test _____

18. knows what a normal temperature is
    (and can tell you) _____

19. exercises at least 3 times a week _____

20. loves chocolate chip cookies _____

Conversation
(pair activity)

With a partner, read or respond to the following. Then change roles and repeat the process. Be sure that your partner makes the correct choice.

PARTNER A

1. Mark is trying out for the basketball team. He needs a physical.
2. The doctor is examining Mark. He is asking him questions at the same time.
3. The doctor examines Mark's eyes and ears. Then he takes Mark's blood pressure.
4. Mark takes a hearing test. He waits to hear a tone. Then he raises his hand.
5. Mark is healthy. He must still get a physical examination.

6. If Mark does not get a physical examination, he cannot be on the basketball team.

7. First Mark must get a physical examination. Then he can enroll at his new school.

PARTNER B

1. a. He needs a *physical* unless he is trying out for the basketball team.

   b. He needs a physical *because* he is trying out for the basketball team.

2. a. The doctor is asking Mark questions *although* he is examining him.

   b. The doctor is asking Mark questions *while* he is examining him.

3. a. The doctor takes Mark's blood pressure *after* he examines Mark's eyes and ears.

   b. The doctor takes Mark's blood pressure *before* he examines Mark's eyes and ears.

4. a. During his hearing test, Mark waits *until* he hears a tone and then he raises his hand.

   b. During his hearing test, Mark waits *although* he hears a tone and then he raises his hand.

5. a. *Although* Mark is healthy, he must get a physical examination anyway.

   b. *Unless* Mark is healthy, he must get a physical examination anyway.

6. a. *Unless* Mark gets a physical examination, he cannot be on the basketball team.

   b. *Because* Mark gets a physical examination, he cannot be on the basketball team.

7. a. Mark can enroll at his new school *before* he gets a physical examination.

   b. Mark can enroll at his new school *after* he gets a physical examination.

15 Childhood Diseases

WORD LIST

Things
childhood diseases
chicken pox
rash
contagious
bumps
calamine lotion
lifetime
contact
measles
spots
fluid
mumps
bedrest

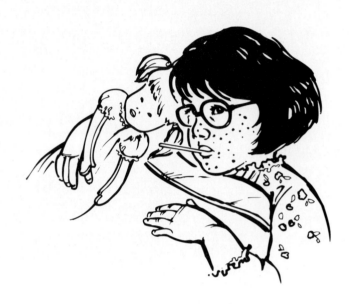

Actions
itch
appear
disappear

Descriptions
awful
infected
persistent

It's Friday afternoon and everybody is looking forward to the weekend—everybody except Cathy. She has chicken pox and she feels awful. She has a fever and a rash and she itches all over.

Cathy didn't go to school today or yesterday and she probably won't go all next week. She's very contagious. She can't see anyone except her mother and father for at least seven days after the red bumps appear.

Usually children younger than Cathy get chicken pox, but a girl at her school didn't stay home when she was contagious and several other kids got chicken pox. It's good Cathy is staying home even though her parents have to miss some work.

For the fever, she takes a non-aspirin drug. Young children shouldn't take aspirin. For the itching, her mother puts calamine lotion on the red bumps and tells Cathy, "Don't scratch them." Scratching may make the bumps bleed and get infected. For the discomfort of being sick, Cathy sleeps and reads books. The good news is that chicken pox only comes once in a lifetime.

Comprehension Check

Circle the correct answer.

1. Cathy feels _____.

   a. fever   b. rash   c. awful

2. Why isn't Cathy going to school next week?

   a. she's contagious   b. children younger than Cathy usually get
                                    chicken pox

   c. her parents have chicken pox

3. What is Cathy taking for her fever?

   a. aspirin   b. a non-aspirin drug

   c. calamine lotion

4. Cathy is using _____ for her itching.

   a. a non-aspirin drug   b. aspirin

   c. calamine lotion

5. Scratching the red bumps can make them _____.

   a. infected   b. go away   c. sleep

6. How many times can you get chicken pox?

   a. once   b. more than once

More Information

Contagious diseases spread by contact with a sick person. You cannot get sick by going outside with wet hair or getting caught in the rain. If children are sick, they shouldn't go to school. If they do, other children may get sick.

The following are other contagious childhood diseases to watch for:

○ *Measles*—Measles begins like a cold. Then red and white spots appear in the mouth, and soon after, a dark red rash on the skin. Measles is contagious one week before the rash as well as during the rash. Give a non-aspirin drug to young children for fever, lots of fluid to drink, and have them rest in a dark room. Watch for persistent fever. Children should be immunized at 15 months.

○ *Mumps*—Mumps begins with a sore throat and a fever, then swelling appears under one or both ears. Mumps is contagious seven days before the swelling and until the swelling disappears. Give a non-aspirin drug to young children for fever, fluids to drink, and bedrest. Children should be immunized.

○ *Strep Throat*—Strep throat is very contagious and needs a doctor's care. It begins with high fever, sore throat, and swelling in the neck. Give a non-aspirin drug to young children for fever, and give an antibiotic.

True or False

Answer with true or false.

1. _____ You can get sick from going outside with wet hair.
2. _____ Parents shouldn't send a child to school if he is sick.
3. _____ Chicken pox are red bumps on the skin.
4. _____ Chicken pox makes you itch a lot.
5. _____ A person with measles should rest in a dark room.
6. _____ Measles usually starts with red and white spots in the mouth.
7. _____ Children should be immunized for measles at ten months.
8. _____ Mumps always cause swelling under both ears.
9. _____ There is no immunization for mumps.
10. _____ Mumps is contagious before you see the swelling.
11. _____ A child who has strep throat should see a doctor.
12. _____ Young children should take aspirin for fever.

Crossword Puzzle

Fill in the words from the word list below.

spots
itch
rash
appear
childhood diseases
contact
disappear
calamine lotion
bumps
awful
lifetime
bedrest
chicken pox
measles
persistent
contagious

ACROSS

1. for example: measles, mumps, and chicken pox
5. when you spread your illness to someone else you are _____
7. red-dot like marks on the skin
9. something that will not go away
11. the time between birth and death
13. the doctor says when you are sick you cannot go to school, you cannot go out to play, you have to stay on _____
14. come into view

DOWN

1. one of the diseases you get as a child—not the measles or mumps
2. when you feel really bad, you feel _____
3. lots of red spots on the skin that may itch
4. a lotion you put on your rash to stop itching
6. the opposite of 14 across
8. to touch someone or something
10. one of the childhood diseases—not the mumps or chicken pox
12. you scratch when you _____
13. a rash can look like _____

Grammar 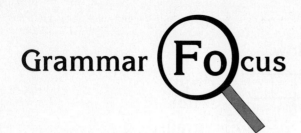 Focus

Contractions

Contractions can combine verbs and their subjects.

> *For example:* it's = it is
> she's = she is
> they'll = they will

Fill in the blanks in the following sentences with contractions.

> *For example:* (It is) _____ Friday afternoon.
> It's Friday afternoon.

1. (It is) _____ good Cathy is staying home.
2. (Cathy is) _____ not in school today.
3. (I am) _____ taking a non-aspirin drug.
4. (She is) _____ very contagious.
5. For the itching, (he is) _____ putting calamine lotion on the red bumps.
6. (They are) _____ leaving at 6:00 A.M.
7. (Mark is) _____ not at home right now.
8. (We are) _____ in the same class she is.

What about you?

- ❍ What childhood diseases have you had?
- ❍ What childhood diseases have your children had?

PRACTICE EXERCISES

Present Tense, Third Person

(pair or individual activity)

Write the verbs in the following sentences in the correct form of the present tense.

Example: Cathy (have) <u>has</u> a contagious disease.

It (**1. be**) _____ Sunday afternoon. The children

(**2. be**) _____ at the park, playing on the swings.

Suddenly Juanita (**3. say**) _____ that she

(**4. do not**) _____ _____ feel good.

She (**5. tell**) _____ her mother that her throat

(**6. hurt**) _____ Her mother (**7. feel**) _____

her forehead and her forearms. They (**8. feel**) _____

very hot. Juanita (**9. put**) _____ her hands up

underneath her ears.

"What (**10. be**) _____ this, Mommy?" she

(**11. ask**) _____, feeling a large lump beneath one

of her ears.

"We'd better call the doctor," her mother (**12. answer**)

_____.

Juanita (**13. go**) _____ home with her mother,

and her mother (**14. call**) _____ the doctor. Then

they (**15. go**) _____ to see the doctor.

The doctor (**16. examine**) _____ Juanita and

(**17. decide**) _____ that she has mumps.

Juanita (**18. have**) _____ to stay at home in bed

for a week. Her mother (**19. give**) _____ her a non-

aspirin drug for discomfort. Juanita's mother really

(**20. wish**) _____ she had had Juanita immunized

against mumps. Too late now!

Tag Questions
(pair activity)

Take one part in the following dialogue, and fill in the proper words for the tag questions.

    Example: A: Cathy has the chicken pox.
                 B: She should stay home from school, <u>shouldn't</u> she?

A: Everybody is looking forward to this weekend except Cathy.

B: I was wondering about her. She didn't go to school today, _____ _____?

A: No, she has chicken pox. That's a contagious disease, _____ _____?

B: Yes, it is. You weren't near her recently, _____ _____?

A: Unfortunately I was. You don't think I'll catch it, _____ _____?

B: Let's hope not, but you'd better watch out for the symptoms. You know what they are, _____ _____?

A: I think you get a fever and some bumps that itch a lot. You don't know of any other symptoms, _____ _____?

B: No, but I know you're not supposed to scratch those itchy bumps or they will leave scars. Cathy isn't scratching them, _____ _____?

A: No, her mom is putting calamine lotion on the bumps to stop the itching. I feel sorry for her, _____ _____?

B: Yes, I do. Surely there is something we can do for her, _____ _____?

A: We could get her a "get well" card, and maybe a book to read. You know what she likes to read, _____ _____?

B: I think I could find something she would like. You will help me look, _____ _____?

A: Sure. Let's go now. Say, I just remembered. I've already had chicken pox. I can't get it again, _____ _____?

B: No, so you don't have to worry about giving her the card and book, _____ _____?

Contagious Diseases

(pair activity)

Ask your partner for the information for your blank boxes. Use the conversation below. Write the information in your boxes. Partner B's chart is in Appendix A, page 227. *Do not look at your partner's page.*

PARTNER A

A: What is/are _____'s _____?

B: His/Her _____ is/are _____.

Name	Symptoms	Disease	Treatment
Ivan	sore throat, swelling under one ear		bedrest, drink fluids, non-aspirin drug
Susanna		strep throat	
Irene		chicken pox	bedrest, calamine lotion, non-aspirin drug
David	red and white spots in mouth, dark red skin rash, fever		

16

Lice

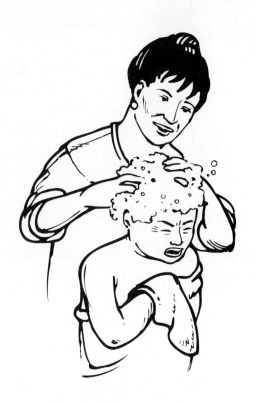

WORD LIST

Things
lice
scalp
nits
hairline
insect
directions
fine-tooth comb
bed linens
nurse
furniture

Actions
scratch
remove
jump
fly
spread

Cathy is at home after school playing with a friend. Theresa notices that she's scratching her head a lot.

Three days later Cathy brings a note home from school about lice. The note says that a few children from Cathy's class have lice. It says that the first symptom of lice is persistent scratching of the scalp. The note also tells parents to check their children for:

1. Tiny white nits that are difficult to remove on the hair close to the scalp

2. Lice in the hair close to the scalp.

3. A rash on the hairline or neck

Theresa is worried, but she wants Tomas to check Cathy's scalp. "I can't stand insects," she says.

Tomas finds nits in Cathy's hair and he thinks he sees something move, but he isn't sure.

Right away he buys some special shampoo and a fine-tooth comb, as the note suggests, and the whole family washes their hair according to the directions because lice are very contagious.

"I can't stand the smell of this stuff!" says Mark. But no one listens.

Tomas carefully combs Cathy's hair with the fine-tooth comb to remove the nits. And Theresa washes Cathy's bed linens and all the combs and brushes in the house in very hot water.

Cathy is upset. "I can't stand lice! Does this mean I'm dirty, Mom?" she wants to know.

"Of course not, dear. Anyone can get lice, but only from a person who has them."

Comprehension Check

Circle the correct answer.

1. What does Cathy bring home from school?

   a. a note about lice   b. a few children   c. special shampoo

2. The first symptom of lice is _____.

   a. a rash   b. a fever   c. persistent scratching of the scalp

3. What doesn't Tomas buy?

   a. a fine-tooth comb   b. bed linens   c. special shampoo

4. Why does the whole family wash their hair?

   a. because lice are very contagious   b. because they have dirty hair

   c. because the shampoo smells good

5. Only people who are dirty get lice.

   a. true   b. false

Cultural Note

Anyone can get lice, but most often young children get them at school, and family members get them from their children. The school nurse will check children about twice a year. Parents should not send a child to school if he or she has lice. Lice are very contagious.

Most lice are on people because lice need blood and hair to live. Lice do not live on animals, furniture, or in carpets. Lice do not jump or fly. And lice do not spread diseases.

Word Search

Circle the following words in the puzzle. Words go across and down.

INSECTS	FLY	SCALP	BED LINENS
PERSISTENT	SCRATCH	LICE	SPREAD
NURSE	REMOVE	FINE-TOOTH	HAIRLINE
NITS	JUMP	COMBS	

```
S C A L P A B O Y A P A C F B O E H J
P C R L E M Q S T Y V P D I A E T C W
R W M Y R O Q G R L B Q I N S E C T S
E B H E S C R A T C H I A E R C L I L
A U D E I B U C E S T R M T I C H K S
D A E C S E T R I E V E Y O D T A A Y
U F S E T A F L Y Z U M S O H O I L E
L D Y O E P E V E G N O P T E N R C L
I E H R N U R S E W S V I H L P L R I
C I V U T P F T I X S E K C L E I M X
E G T A P E D M L T J R Y O R D N S E
A E S E K D R A W R Z S N M R U E R L
T H R W E L M E N E T M A B F R N I K
N I T S M B E D L I N E N S N J U M P
```

Matching

Match the word with the meaning.

1. _____ what you do when you itch
2. _____ a tiny insect that lives in your hair
3. _____ for example: sheets, blankets, and pillowcases
4. _____ for example: sofa, table, and chairs
5. _____ go from one person to another
6. _____ to take away
7. _____ used to remove lice from the hair
8. _____ the part of the head where hair grows
9. _____ lice are a type of _____
10. _____ follow the _____ to do it right

a. bed linens
b. spread
c. remove
d. scratch
e. fine-tooth comb
f. lice
g. scalp
h. insect
i. directions
j. furniture

Grammar Focus

Use of "can't stand"

Use "can't stand" to express strong dislike.

For example: I can't stand broccoli.

List three things you can't stand.

1. _____.
2. _____.
3. _____.

List three things your partner can't stand. (Ask your partner, "What can't you stand?")

For example: He <u>can't</u> <u>stand</u> dogs.

1. _____.
2. _____
3. _____

PRACTICE EXERCISES

Pronunciation Exercise

(pair activity)

Copy the following lists of words (Partner A's are listed here. Partner B's are in Appendix A, pages 228-229). Where it says "Listen and check" put a check mark by the word your partner pronounces. Where it says "Pronounce" say the word that is underlined, and your partner will put a check mark by that word. *Do not look at your partner's page.* When you are finished, correct your answers. If you don't know how to pronounce a word, ask the teacher.

PARTNER A

1. Listen and check:

   hair _____

   here _____

   higher _____

2. Pronounce:

   lice

   lies

   <u>rice</u>

3. Listen and check:

   dirty _____

   thirty _____

   ditty _____

4. Pronounce:

   nerds

   <u>Norse</u>

   nurse

5. Listen and check:

   escape _____

   scalp _____

   scald _____

6. Pronounce:

   <u>back in the
     station</u>

   vaccination

   vacation

7. Listen and check:

   hate _____

   height _____

   high _____

8. Pronounce:

   buys

   vice

   <u>bites</u>

9. Listen and check:

   rash _____

10. Pronounce:

    <u>blush</u>

lash	_____	bush	
rush	_____	brush	

11. Listen and check:

spread _____

sprayed _____

sprit _____

12. Pronounce:

<u>scratch</u>

scrap

scrapes

13. Listen and check:

fly _____

flea _____

flew _____

14. Pronounce:

head

<u>hid</u>

heed

Vocabulary Match-Up

Your teacher will give you a slip of paper with one of the following items. Find the person whose slip matches the word or definition on your slip of paper.

scalp	○ tables, chairs, sofas, etc.
lice	○ a short written letter
first symptom of lice	○ able to be caught by some one else
remove	○ floor covering
dirty	○ what you do when something itches
fine-tooth comb	○ insects that live on human hair and blood
contagious	○ not clean
bed linens	○ persistent scratching of the scalp
note	○ the skin on the top and back of the head
scratch	○ used to remove nits
carpet	○ to take away, to take out of
furniture	○ sheets and pillowcases

Role Play

Act out the following situations in groups of 3, 4, or 5. Be sure that everyone has something to say.

1. Two people are in the restroom in front of the mirror. One asks the other if he/she can borrow a brush. A guardian angel appears to warn of the dangers of catching head lice from someone else's brush. A devil also appears and says it's O.K. to borrow someone else's brush. What do the two people decide to do?

2. A parent takes his/her children to the doctor. The doctor's nurse discovers that the children have head lice. What questions do the children and the parent ask the doctor? What does the doctor tell them to do? What does the doctor prescribe?

3. Three friends are talking together. One starts scratching his/her head a lot. How do the other two politely suggest that maybe someone should check for head lice?

4. A person is at the pharmacy getting the prescription shampoo for head lice. The pharmacist is hard of hearing. How do other customers react when they hear the customer's request and the pharmacist's instructions? What do the other customers say?

5. Three nits are talking to each other about how they got where they are, how they like it there, and where they are going to go next. Then along comes Mr. Hasta La Vista Baby Shampoo to spoil all their fun.

6. A parent is explaining to the family what must be done with bed linens, brushes, and combs in the house because they have lice. Also, the children will have to stay home from school for a day or two. The children are upset. How does the parent make them understand that they are not "dirty" and that everything will be O.K.?

Smoking

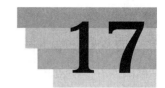

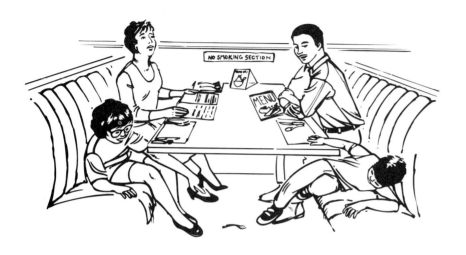

17

WORD LIST

Things
smoking
hostess
nonsmoking section
lung cancer
heart disease
risk
pregnancy
miscarriage
restriction
policy
research
private organization
acquaintance

Descriptions
proud
premature
especially

It's Friday night and the Santos family is going out to dinner. Theresa feels a little tired because she's had her new job only two weeks. But now they have more money to go out to eat. Mark feels a little impatient because he's going to a school dance after dinner and they're eating late. Cathy is a little excited because her father has been telling her what a special dinner this is. But Tomas is very excited! He has been looking forward to this evening for nearly a month. And he wants to share it with his family.

In fact, he almost didn't let Mark go to the dance. Tomas tells the hostess, "A table for four, please—nonsmoking." This is the first time they have been out to eat and sat in the non-smoking section of a restaurant. He feels proud of himself. He hasn't smoked for one month. Now the doctor will be happier with his pulse. Tomas will be safer from lung cancer and heart disease.

143

And his family won't be at risk from breathing smoke. He also knows that children get habits from their parents. They'll all be healthier. Besides, Tomas is thinking about the baby he and Theresa want. He knows that mothers who smoke or breathe smoke during pregnancy have more miscarriages and more premature babies than mothers who do not breathe smoke.

Tomas is happy to be with his family tonight and he is especially happy they are all healthy. They are happy too, but Tomas is the happiest.

Comprehension Check

Circle the correct answer.

1. Who is the happiest member of the Santos family tonight?

   a. Theresa   b. Mark   c. Tomas

2. Where does Tomas want to sit in the restaurant?

   a. the smoking section   b. the nonsmoking section

3. Why is Tomas so proud?

   a. He stopped smoking.   b. It's his birthday.

   c. Theresa is going to have a baby.

4. Tomas is happy only for himself about not smoking.

   a. true   b. false

 # Cultural Note

All over America we see more and more restrictions on smoking. For example, all airlines have a no-smoking policy during flights within the United States. Also, more and more restaurants and public places have nonsmoking sections.

One reason for this is that research is showing that nonsmokers who are around smokers are at as much health risk as smokers, so people don't want to be near smokers. Another reason is that more and more diseases are being found to be caused by smoking. Smoking causes one out of every six deaths in the United States.

According to the Surgeon General, every day more than 3,000 teenagers in the United States begin to smoke. But almost half of all adults who once smoked have quit since 1965. Smoking is expensive, too. The average smoker smokes 34 cigarettes a day at a cost of $1,200 per year.

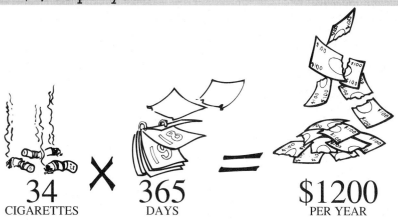

34	X	365	=	$1200
CIGARETTES		DAYS		PER YEAR

Help for people who want to stop smoking is available from a doctor, the American Cancer Society, and Smokers Anonymous. While private organizations give stop-smoking classes that can be expensive, local hospitals offer inexpensive or free classes for smokers.

Fill in the Blank

Fill in the blanks with the correct words from the word list below.

policy   pregnancy
risk   research
premature   lung cancer
miscarriage   heart disease
smoking   nonsmoking sections

One out of every six deaths in the U.S. is caused by

(1) _____. The (2) _____ of diseases

like (3) _____ _____ and

(4) _____ _____ is much greater

among smokers. (5) _____ shows that women

have some special risks. During (6) _____ the risk

of having a (7) _____ or a (8) _____

baby is greater among women who smoke or breathe someone else's smoke. For these reasons, all airlines have a no smoking (9) _____ during flights within the U.S. Also, restaurants and public buildings have (10) _____

_____.

Grammar 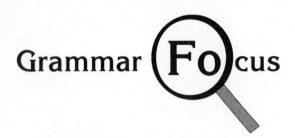cus

Comparatives

Use "-er" or "more" + "than" to compare two things.
Use "-er" + "than" with words of one syllable or with words ending in "y."

For example: Spring is cool<u>er</u> <u>than</u> summer.
The smoking section is smok<u>ier</u> <u>than</u> the nonsmoking section.

(*Note:* The "y" changes to "i" before adding the ending.)
Use "more" + "than" with words of two or more syllables (except those ending in y).

For example: Running is <u>more</u> difficult <u>than</u> walking.

Write the correct comparative form in each blank.

For example: Mark is (old) _____ Cathy.
Mark is <u>older</u> <u>than</u> Cathy.

or

Tomas is (excited) _____ his family.
Tomas is <u>more</u> <u>excited</u> <u>than</u> his family.

1. Theresa is (tired) _____ Tomas.
2. Tomas is (healthy) _____ he was before he quit smoking.
3. Ice is (cold) _____ than water.
4. Tomas is (happy) _____ before he quit smoking.

5. She quit smoking (soon) _____ we expected.

6. A nonsmoker is (safe) _____ from lung cancer

_____ a smoker.

>   (*Note:* In this sentence, "*than*" is separated from the comparative.)

7. Some people think vegetables are (delicious) _____ meat.

8. Fruit is (economical) _____ than cigarettes.

What about you?

- ❍ Are you a smoker?
- ❍ If you're a smoker, who breathes your smoke?
- ❍ If you aren't a smoker, do you breathe smoke?
- ❍ If you don't like smoke and an acquaintance comes to your house and says, "Do you mind if I smoke?" what do you say?
- ❍ If you're sitting in the nonsmoking section of a restaurant and someone starts smoking, do you ask him/her to stop?
- ❍ Do Americans feel differently about smoking than people in your country?

———— PRACTICE EXERCISES ————

Conversation
(pair activity)

Partner A will start the following conversation (#1). Partner B must then decide which response (#2, a or b) is appropriate. Partner A will then respond with the appropriate response (#3, a or b) to Partner B, and so on. The conversation will not make sense unless the correct choices are made.

PARTNER A

1. Did you see the Santos family at the restaurant last night? Theresa looked a little tired.

3. a. Yes, he did. I wonder if he was going to the school dance after dinner. Do you think that's it?

b. No, they aren't. But what did you tell that old man who was smoking in the corner? Was he bothering you?

5. a. No, they wouldn't. Smoking bothers them too much. It bothers me, too. I'm glad they put in a nonsmoking section, aren't you?

   b. He certainly did. But I think he was even prouder of being able to sit in the nonsmoking section. Have you heard that he quit smoking?

PARTNER B

2. a. I wouldn't eat there. The hostess is nice, but they don't have a nonsmoking section, do they?

   b. Yes, she did, but she's still getting used to her new job. Mark looked anxious about something, didn't he?

4. a. That's probably it. Didn't Tomas look proud to have his whole family out together for dinner at a restaurant?

   b. He told the hostess they wanted a table for four in the nonsmoking section. Did they get it?

6. a. Sometimes. But I think they should change it.

   b. Yes, for over a month now. I think that's great.

Choral Reading: Song

The following should be sung to the tune of "On Top of Old Smoky." Try to pick up the rhythm of the words. This will help your intonation and pronunciation.

Joe once was a smoker
All filled with regret;
His false-hearted lover
Was his cigarette.

He wanted her with him
All places he went
But others despised her
And that awful scent.

In restaurants they told him
She couldn't come in
On airplanes they banned her
And all of her kin.

Joe's family begged him,
"Get rid of her quick!"
Her heady aroma
Had made them all sick.

But Joe wouldn't leave her
He craved her so much
She told him she loved him
And warmed to his touch.

Now false-hearted lovers
Can bring you down low
It's better to leave them
And then "just say no."

Joe quit her "cold turkey"
On Thanksgiving Day
And so far he's grateful
That she's stayed away.

So come all you smokers
There's hope for you yet;
It's time you discarded
That last cigarette.

Find Someone in the Class Who . . .

1. has never smoked a cigarette _____

2. has tried cigarettes but didn't like them _____

3. has smoked cigarettes for more than a year _____

4. has wanted to quit smoking but hasn't
   quit yet _____

5. has successfully quit smoking _____

6. has known someone who died of
   lung cancer _____

7. has asked a smoker to put out his/her
   cigarette _____

8. has requested a nonsmoking section
   in a restaurant   _____
9. has tried a stop-smoking class   _____
10. has lived with a smoker   _____

Art Project

In groups of 3 or 4, create posters that advocate either quitting smoking or smokers' rights. On the back of the poster, list at least three arguments in favor of your position. Be prepared to defend your views to the rest of the class.

Alcohol

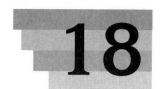

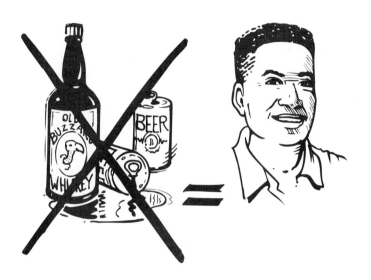

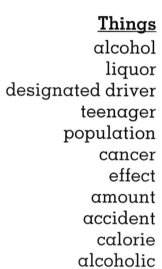

18

Things

alcohol
liquor
designated driver
teenager
population
cancer
effect
amount
accident
calorie
alcoholic

Descriptions

uncomfortable
loudly
strange
designated
common

popular
long term
dangerous
seldom
drunk

Mark gets home from the restaurant with his family just as his friends come to pick him up to go to the dance.

"Bye, Mom. Bye, Dad," he says quickly. And he's out the door. He doesn't want to hear again all the things he's supposed to do and not do.

In the car with his friends he feels as though he can be more himself. He feels that what he says is important.

In the parking lot when they get to the school, one of his friends takes a bottle of liquor out from under the seat. He has a big smile. Both his friends take a drink from the bottle and one says, "Here Mark, it's your turn."

Mark wants his friends to like him, but he feels uncomfortable. "I . . . I don't really feel like it," he says and gets out of the car. But his friends don't follow him.

He doesn't see them until the dance is almost over. When he talks to them they seem strange, not like friends at all.

Mark isn't sure what to do. He knows he shouldn't ride home with them. It's late, but he decides to call his father for a ride. "He'll probably be angry and not let me go out for a while," Mark thinks as he goes outside to wait, "but it's better than driving home with someone who's been drinking."

But when Mark's father comes he isn't angry. He tells Mark he was right to call. "I'm proud of you, son," he says, "and in a couple of years when you're old enough to drive remember when you go out always to have a designated driver who won't drink."

"Dad," says Mark, "Can we take Bill and John home too so they don't drive?"

Comprehension Check

Circle the correct answer.

1. Where is Mark going with his friends?

   a. to a restaurant   b. to a parking lot   c. to a dance

2. Mark is in a hurry to leave for the dance with his friends.

   a. true   b. false

3. What do Mark's friends want him to do?

   a. drink alcohol   b. go to a party   c. drive them home

4. How does Mark feel when his friends start drinking?

   a. He feels important.   b. He feels uncomfortable.

   c. He feels O.K.

5. When Mark's friends have too much to drink, he decides
   to _____.

   a. call his father for a ride home   b. make his friends dance

   c. take their alcohol away

6. Mark doesn't want his friends to _____.

   a. meet his father   b. drive themselves home   c. dance

Cultural Note

Use of alcohol is common among teenagers, and it is more common than ever now that other drugs are becoming less popular. The U.S. Department of Health and Human Services says that over half of all teenagers drink at least once a month. Parents, again, set the example. About two-thirds of the adult population drink at least sometimes.

The health risks of long term heavy use of alcohol are great. It is the third greatest cause of death in the United States after cancer and heart disease. Alcohol also destroys vitamins and has lots of calories.

But the immediate risk of driving after drinking may be the most important because this affects everyone on the road. Even small amounts of alcohol can dangerously affect driving ability. Many, many deaths (25,000 a year) in auto accidents occur because drivers think they can drive just as well after drinking alcohol. In fact, one out of every two traffic deaths is alcohol-related.

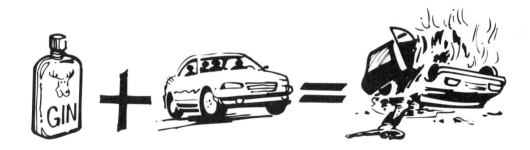

Like pregnant women who smoke, pregnant women who drink alcohol (even one or two glasses a day) have more miscarriages and premature babies than other women.

The annual expense due to alcohol use, in accidents, property damage, lost work time, health care, and insurance is $117 billion a year.

Someone who gets drunk often or who depends on alcohol to get through the day is an alcoholic. Many teenagers drink to gain a feeling of importance because they think no one cares about them. Teenagers who feel loved by their parents seldom become alcoholics. But there are free programs such as Al-Anon and Alateen to help alcoholics of all ages. Call your local health department for information.

Crossword Puzzle

Fill in the words from the word list below.

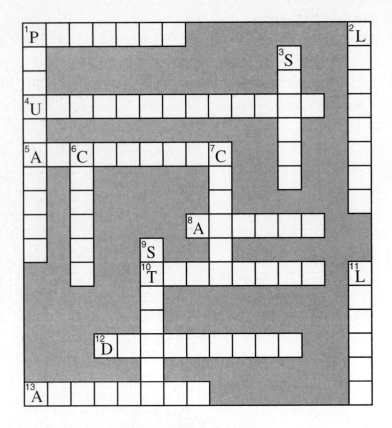

common
liquor
alcoholic
teenager
accident
popular
seldom
population
long-term
cancer
strange
amount
dangerous
uncomfortable

ACROSS

1. when most people like something it is _____
4. when you don't feel good about something
5. a person who cannot stop drinking alcohol
8. even a small _____ of alcohol can be dangerous when driving
10. a person older than 12 but younger than 20
12. it is very _____ to drink and drive
13. if you drink and drive you may have an _____

DOWN

1. the people who live in a place
2. the opposite of short-term
3. the opposite of often
6. a leading cause of death from disease
7. used often
9. unusual or different
11. beer, wine, and brandy are examples of _____

Grammar 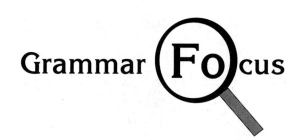cus

Negatives with "don't" and "doesn't"

Use the contractions "don't" and "doesn't" to make negative sentences in the present tense.

For example: don't = do not
doesn't = does not

For example: I <u>don't</u> have any money.

or

He <u>doesn't</u> like big cities.

(*Note:* Do not add "s" or "es" at the end of the main verb in the third-person singular present tense. The verbs "do" or "does" show the agreement.)

Make negative sentences using "don't" and "doesn't" from the following affirmative sentences.

For example: His friends follow him.
<u>His</u> <u>friends</u> <u>don't</u> <u>follow</u> <u>him</u>.

1. He sees them when the dance is over.

   He _____.

2. Mark takes a drink from the bottle.

   Mark _____.

3. I really feel like drinking.

   I _____.

4. She calls on Sundays.

   She _____.

5. They drive.

   They _____.

6. Mark calls his father for a ride home.

   Mark _____.

7. We feel comfortable.

We _____.

8. Maria speaks English.

Maria _____.

What about you?

○ Do you drink before driving?

○ If you have children, do you set a good example for them?

○ If you have children, do they know where they can get a ride if they are with a driver who has been drinking?

○ Do you know anyone who is an alcoholic and needs help?

━━━ PRACTICE EXERCISES ━━━

Interview
(pair activity)

Ask your partner the following questions and write down your partner's answers. Be prepared to present your findings to the class.

1. How do you feel about insects? Are there some you dislike more than others?

   _____.

2. What can you say to someone who wants to borrow your hairbrush?

   _____.

3. What would you say to someone who was blowing cigarette smoke in your face?

   _____.

4. How do you feel about pregnant women who smoke?

   _____.

5. What is meant by the term "designated driver"?

   _____.

6. Your best friend is drunk and wants to drive home. What do you do?

   _____.

7. If you owned a restaurant, how would you feel about non-smoking sections?

_____.

8. How would you stop a teenager from trying his/her first cigarette?

_____.

9. Have you ever known an alcoholic? Describe this person.

_____.

10. How do advertisements encourage the use of alcohol in our country?

_____.

Negatives
(pair activity)

Listen and choose the correct answer as your partner asks you questions. Only one of the choices is grammatically correct. Ask your partner questions and make sure that you both agree on which answer is correct.

PARTNER A	PARTNER B
1. Listen and answer: No, he don't have no time to change his clothes. No, he doesn't have no time to change his clothes. No, he doesn't have any time to change his clothes.	**1. Ask:** When Mark gets home, does he change his clothes for the dance?
2. Ask: Is he supposed to clean his room before he leaves?	**2. Listen and answer:** No, he ain't. No, he isn't. No, he wasn't.
3. Listen and answer: No, he couldn't. No, he can't. No, he didn't.	**3. Ask:** Could he feel more like himself when he was with his family?

PARTNER A (continued)

4. Ask:

Does Mark have a bottle of liquor with him?

5. Listen and answer:

No, he couldn't.

No, he can't.

No, he didn't.

6. Ask:

Have you ever been drunk?

7. Listen and answer:

No, I won't never drink and drive.

No, I wouldn't ever drink and drive.

No, I wouldn't never drink and drive.

PARTNER B (continued)

4. Listen and answer:

No, he doesn't have a bottle

No, he don't have a bottle.

No, he doesn't have no bottle.

5. Ask:

Can he go home immediately?

6. Listen and answer:

No, I haven't never been drunk.

No, I ain't ever been drunk.

No, I haven't ever been drunk.

7. Ask:

Would you ever drink and drive?

Dice Game

(group activity)

Taking turns, roll a die and move the number of spaces shown. If you land on an empty square, stay there and wait for your next turn. If you land on a square with a sentence, say whether it is correct or incorrect. If it is incorrect, correct it. If you are right, move ahead two squares. If you are incorrect, move back two squares.

FINISH 50	A designated driver can only have 3 beers at a party. 49	Pregnant women should avoid alcohol. 48	47	U.S. airlines have a no smoking policy. 46
41	Secondary smoke can be harmful to children. 42	43	Smokers Anonymous urges teenagers to smoke. 44	45
"Proud" rhymes with "crowd." 40	39	"I don't want no drink" is correct English. 38	37	"Seldom" means "not very often." 36
31	A scalp is the inside of the lung. 32	33	34	"Lice" rhymes with "lease." 35
30	29	Only very dirty people get lice. 28	27	Lice are not very contagious. 26
I **have**; Juan **haves**. 22		A symptom of strep throat is red spots on the skin. 24	25	
Calamine lotion is used on the red bumps of mumps. 11	Children should take aspirin for fever during chicken pox. 19	18	For measles, you should rest in a dark room. 17	16
10		"Physical" rhymes with "bicycle." 13	14	Today you **tell**; yesterday you **telled**. 15
START 1	Students in the U.S. do not need vaccinations for school. 9	You may need a tetanus shot if you step on a rusty nail. 8	7	"Slight" means "a lot." 6
	Pneumonia is a respiratory disease. 2	3	He **goes**; He **went**; He **has went**. 4	Your "pulse" is your heartbeat. 5

19

Drugs

WORD LIST

Things
parade
band
flag
sign
speech
country
education
rehabilitation
addict
mind
crime
truth
pill
energy
reason
capsule
attitude
jail
career

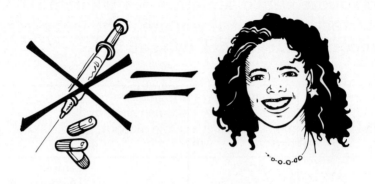

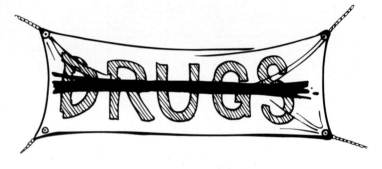

Actions
wave
recover
wonder
tear
ruin

Descriptions
lonely
sad
miserable
informed
concerned

Today there is a parade downtown, but it isn't a holiday. Six schools are participating in a "Say No to Drugs" parade. The high school bands are playing in uniform and cheerleaders are waving colorful flags. The kids from Cathy's school are carrying signs saying "Get High on Life, not Drugs." Even the mayor is going to give a speech.

This city and many others across the country are very concerned about drugs in schools. At Mark's school, the parade is part of a whole drug education program with speakers from a drug rehabilitation center, talks by recovered addicts, and movies.

Why is everyone so concerned? Maybe it's because drugs affect people's minds and bodies in so many ways, and no one completely understands the effects. Maybe it's because drugs often go with crime. Maybe it's because people are afraid teenagers will try anything and don't know the dangers.

Cathy understands that people get very upset about drugs, but she doesn't know why. Today she's thinking more about the flags and the band.

Mark wonders if adults tell the truth about how bad drugs are. Some kids at school say they're great. Today he's thinking more about not going to school because he's in the parade.

Comprehension Check

Circle the correct answer.

1. Today there is a _____ downtown.

   a. holiday   b. parade   c. drugs

2. The parade is to increase awareness about _____.

   a. cheerleaders   b. flags   c. drugs

3. What are people across the country concerned about?

   a. drugs in schools   b. movies   c. speakers

4. Which one is a concern about drugs?

   a. Drugs go with crime.   b. Drugs affect people many ways.

   c. both a. and b.

5. Cathy understands why people get upset about drugs.

   a. true   b. false

6. Does Mark understand whether drugs are good or bad?

   a. He's sure.   b. He's not sure.

 # Cultural Note

Americans like things to happen quickly. They don't like to wait for anything. If they have a headache, they take a pill to make it disappear. If they're tired, they take a pill to give them energy because it's quicker than sleeping. If they have a cold, they take a cold capsule, and on and on and on.

It's no surprise that children get the idea there's a pill for everything—feeling worried, feeling lonely, feeling sad. They learn from the people around them that there's no reason to wait for time to heal their problems when a drug can do it faster.

This attitude leads to the abuse of all kinds of drugs, which kills thousands of people every year and makes life miserable for many more. It tears families apart, puts people in jail, and ruins careers.

But these facts mean little to a teenager who wants to be accepted, or who feels bad and doesn't know how to feel good except with drugs. As with alcohol, teenagers who feel loved seldom turn to drug abuse.

At least if children and teenagers are informed about drugs, they can make better choices for their own lives.

Word Groups

Cross out the word that does *not* belong.

1. band speech flag capsule
2. sign lonely sad miserable
3. recover wave wonder speech
4. attitude mind concerned reason

Matching

Match the word with the meaning.

1. ____ where criminals go   a. band
2. ____ a person who cannot stop
          taking drugs   b. sad
3. ____ a group of musicians   c. to be concerned
4. ____ to care or worry about
          something   d. pill
5. ____ feeling alone   e. jail
6. ____ a tiny ball of medicine   f. career
7. ____ a job you choose   g. crime
8. ____ not happy   h. country
9. ____ illegal act   i. lonely
10. ____ for example: the United States   j. addict

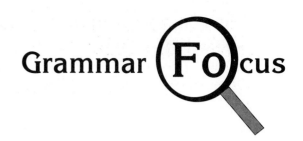

Use of "maybe"

Use "maybe" to give a possible explanation or a possible answer to a question beginning with "why."

For example: Why are people concerned about drugs?
<u>Maybe</u> it's because drugs and crime go together.

Choose an answer for each question from the list below.

drugs lead to crime
it's Friday
it's important to tell people how
  dangerous drugs are

I exercise and I don't smoke
I didn't study
they want a fast answer to their
  problems

1. Why are you so healthy?

   Maybe it's because _____

   _____.

2. Why are you worried about the exam?

   Maybe it's because _____

   _____.

3. Why is everyone so worried about drugs?

   Maybe it's because _____

   _____.

4. Why is everyone so happy?

   Maybe it's because _____

   _____.

5. Why do people take drugs?

   Maybe it's because _____

   _____.

6. Why is there a "Say No to Drugs" parade downtown?

Maybe it's because _____

_____.

Can you ask a "why" question and give an answer?

Why _____?

Maybe it's because _____

_____.

What about you?

- ○ Does talking about drugs upset you?
- ○ If you have children, do you know how they feel about drugs?
- ○ If you have children, do you trust them to make good deci-sions about drugs?
- ○ Do you think people understand the dangers of drugs?

—— PRACTICE EXERCISES ——

Cloze Exercise

(pair or individual activity)

Fill in the blanks with the appropriate word from the word list below. Use each word only once.

ruin	problems	lonely	addicted
restless	people	money	rehabilitation
appetite	recovers	job	miserable
jail			

Jared was having a lot of personal problems. He had no friends to turn to for help. He felt (1) _____ and
(2) _____. He turned to drugs as an escape from
his (3) _____ and before he knew it, he became
(4) _____. He tried to hide his drug habit, but the
(5) _____ who worked with him noticed that his
moods kept changing. One minute he appeared to be tired, but

the next minute he appeared to be (6) _____. He started coming to work late, and then he did a poor (7) _____. He didn't eat much because he had lost his (8) _____. Soon he started not showing up at work at all. Then when he did show up, he always said he was broke and needed (9) _____. One day a policeman came to Jared's place of work and arrested him. Jared was put in (10) _____ for selling drugs. Since this was his first offense, the judge gave him a choice between staying in jail or entering a drug (11) _____ program. Jared chose the rehabilitation program. Let's hope that Jared (12) _____ and that drugs do not (13) _____ the rest of his life.

Negative Commands
(pair activity)

Give your partner the following negative commands:

For example: Tell your partner: not to tell you that you're beautiful
(You say): "<u>Don't</u> <u>tell</u> <u>me</u> <u>that</u> <u>I'm</u> <u>beautiful</u>."

PARTNER A
Tell your partner:

1. not to do drugs
3. not to be so difficult
5. not to say you're yelling when you're not
7. not to say you're lying
9. not to look now, but there's a monkey in the room

PARTNER B
Tell your partner:

2. not to tell you what to do
4. not to yell at you
6. not to lie
8. not to look at you like that
10. not to put you on

Say Yes (to Life): Affirmative Commands
(pair activity)
Give your partner the following affirmative commands:

For example: Tell your partner: to smile; he/she is on Candid Camera.
(You say): "<u>Smile. You're on Candid Camera.</u>"

PARTNER A **Tell your partner:**	PARTNER B **Tell your partner:**
1. to have a nice day 3. to keep trying hard 5. to stay as wonderful as he/she is 7. to let you give him/her a million dollars 9. to say something exciting	2. to take care of himself/herself 4. to keep up the good work 6. to trust you 8. to let you drive him/her to the bank 10. to listen to your wonderful teacher

Small Group Discussion

In groups of 4 or 5, discuss the following issues and write down your group's feelings. Be prepared to report the results to the rest of the class.

1. Why do you think so many young people get addicted to drugs in this country? Name at least three more possible reasons besides the ones already mentioned in Lesson 19.

    1. _____
    2. _____
    3. _____

2. Many people think that television and movies contribute to "glamorizing" the use of drugs. Why do you think they say this? Have you ever seen something in a movie or on television that made drugs look harmless or attractive?

    _____

    _____

    _____

3. What do you think is actually being done to educate our young people about the dangers of drugs? What more could be done?

_____

_____

_____

4. What if there were a drug you could take that would instantly enable you to speak perfect English, but it had the side effect of forcing you to tell the truth at *all* times, even when you would prefer to say nothing. Would you take it?

_____

_____

_____

20 Acquired Immunity Deficiency Syndrome (AIDS)

WORD LIST

Things
AIDS
hall
booklet
virus
sex
drug needle
touch
birth
condom

Actions
notice
miss
catch up
yell
calm down

touch
share
spread

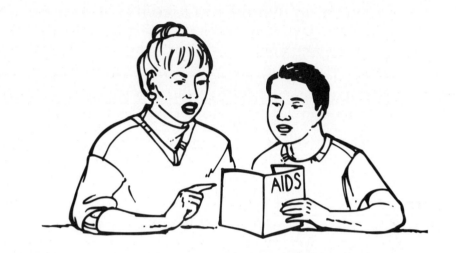

Descriptions
smart
infected

One day three months into the school year a new boy came to Mark's class. Mark noticed that the other kids didn't talk to him much, so Mark started talking to him after class and in the halls. Mark remembered what it was like to be new in school.

After a couple of weeks, they ate lunch together one day in the cafeteria. Mark liked Larry, but found him different from his other friends. Larry liked to read and he didn't play sports.

"Where did you go to school before?" Mark asked. "This is my school," Larry answered. I went here last year and part of this year . . . before I went in the hospital."

"I thought you were new in school. I never saw you until two weeks ago." Mark stopped and then asked, "Why were you in the hospital?"

Larry answered "Well . . . I don't want everyone in school to know, but I have AIDS. By the way, Mark, what's your phone number in case I have a question about any school work I've missed?" Larry said he had a lot of studying to do to catch up.

Mark wondered, "Why does he want to ask *me* about schoolwork!" But he said "Sure," and gave Larry his number. He liked Larry and he knew Larry wanted to be friends.

That evening Mark told his mother about Larry. Theresa was glad Mark had a new friend who was interested in school, but when she heard he had AIDS she got upset and she started yelling at Mark. She was afraid Mark might get AIDS from Larry.

Mark tried to calm his mother down. "There's nothing to worry about," he told her, "I'll show you." And he showed her a booklet he had gotten at school from a public health nurse who had spoken to his class. The booklet said you cannot get AIDS by touching, sharing meals, hugging, swimming, or sharing a bathroom with someone who has AIDS.

Sometimes Mark thinks his mother isn't so smart. But most of all, he feels sad for Larry.

Comprehension Check

Circle the correct answer.

1. Is Larry new in Mark's school?

   a. Yes, he is.   b. No, he isn't.

2. Why does Mark first talk to Larry?

   a. because few students talk to him   b. because Mark has AIDS

   c. because Larry is his friend

3. What does Larry want from Mark?

   a. someone to be friends with   b. his phone number for help with homework

   c. both a and b

Lesson 20   Acquired Immune Deficiency Syndrome (AIDS)   **169**

4. Why is Theresa upset?

    a. because Mark doesn't study   b. because has a new friend

    c. because she's afraid Mark might get AIDS from Larry

5. You cannot get AIDS just from hugging a person with AIDS.

    a. true   b. false

More Information

Acquired Immunity Deficiency Syndrome (AIDS) spreads only by direct contact with the virus.

People who get AIDS get it by:

○ having *unprotected sex with a person who has AIDS
○ sharing a drug needle with someone who has AIDS
○ getting blood from a person with AIDS
○ birth from a mother with AIDS
○ touching the blood of a person who has AIDS
   where you have a cut or sore

You can get more information about AIDS from:

○ the Public Health Service at (800) 342-AIDS
○ your local American Red Cross
○ your doctor
○ your local Public Health Department

You can also get a free AIDS test at your local Public Health Department. You do not have to give your name to get this test.

Matching

Fill in the blank with the letter of the correct word.

You cannot get AIDS from doing these things with someone who has AIDS:

1. ____   2. ____

3. ____   4. ____

a. touching

b. swimming

c. sharing a drug needle

d. hugging

e. having unprotected sex

*unprotected sex = sex without a condom

You can get AIDS from doing these things with someone who has AIDS:

5. ____   6. ____

7. ____   8. ____

f. getting blood

g. sharing a meal

h. birth from a mother with

Multiple Choice

Circle the correct answer.

1. A disease that is spread only by direct contact with the virus.

   AIDS   a cold

2. A space inside a building used to walk from room to room.

   sidewalk   hall

3. If you take drugs through the skin you use a _____.

   spoon   drug needle

4. AIDS is spread only by direct contact with the _____.

   virus   birth

5. A word that means the time you are born.

   birth   booklet

6. The opposite of "fat" is _____.

   pale   thin

7. A word that means to give part of something to someone else.

   share   spread

8. If someone gets a disease from another person, the disease

   _____.

   spreads   shares

9. If someone has little or no color in her face she is _____.

   pale   thin

10. If you are behind, you must _____.

    miss   catch up

Grammar 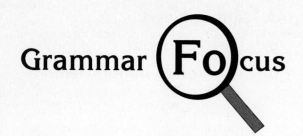cus

"Wh" questions using "where" and "when"

Questions about location often begin with "where."

For example: <u>Where</u> is your school?

Questions about time often begin with "when."

For example: <u>When</u> does your class begin?

Look at the questions and answers below. Fill in each blank with "where" or "when."

For example: Q: _____<u>Where</u>_____ is your school?
A: It's on the corner of B Street and 1st Avenue.

1. Q: _____ did you go to school before?
   A: I went to this school.

2. Q: _____ is your doctor's appointment?
   A: It's at 2:00.

3. Q: _____'s the hospital you're going to?
   A: It's downtown next to the library.

4. Q: _____ can I call for an appointment?
   A: Call after 1 p.m.

5. Q: _____'s your physical examination?
   A: It's next month.

6. Q: _____ did he stop smoking?
   A: He stopped last month.

7. Q: _____'s the best place to go for a flu vaccination?
   A: Go to the county hospital.

8. Q: _____ did you go for your pneumonia vaccination?
   A: I went to the county hospital.

Can you make up a question using "where" and a question using "when"? Can you answer the questions?

Q: Where _____?

A: _____.

Q: When _____?

A: _____.

What about you?

○ Do you know anyone who has AIDS or who died from AIDS?

○ Are you afraid to be friends with someone who has AIDS?

══ PRACTICE EXERCISES ══

Pronunciation Exercise: Past Tense with –ed
(pair activity)

There are three ways to pronounce the "–ed" at the end of past tense verbs, One is like the sound "t" (example: "wished"), one is like "id" (example: "started"), and the third is simply the sound of "d" (example: borrowed). Copy the following chart and then ask your partner how to pronounce the past tense verb forms. Repeat the correct pronunciation and write the verb in the correct column on the verb chart. You have half the information; your partner has the other half. So that you really listen and learn the correct pronunciation, be sure not to look at your partner's chart until after you are finished. Partner B's chart is in Appendix A, pages 229-230.

Partner A's question: How do you pronounce the past tense of _____?

	Present	Past		
		–id	–t	–d
Listen and pronounce	1. care			cared
Ask	2. like			
Listen and pronounce	3. tend	tended		
Ask	4. repeat			
Listen and pronounce	5. finish		finished	
Ask	6. play			
Listen and pronounce	7. miss		missed	

	Present	Past		
		–id	–t	–d
Ask	**8.** decide			
Listen and pronounce	**9.** call			called
Ask	**10.** ask			
Listen and pronounce	**11.** want	wanted		
Ask	**12.** share			
Listen and pronounce	**13.** notice		noticed	
Ask	**14.** yell			
Listen and pronounce	**15.** learn			learned
Ask	**16.** wait			
Listen and pronounce	**17.** touch		touched	

Continuous Line Drill

(group activity—review)

Your teacher will tell half the class to write one of the following verbs on a piece of paper. Those people will form an outside circle in the classroom. The other half of the class will form an inside circle facing the outside circle. When the teacher says "Start" the people on the inside will move from one outside person to the next. They must pronounce and spell the **past tense** of each verb. When everyone has gone around the circle twice, the inside circle will take the cards of the outside circle, and the same process will be repeated.

For Example: <u>On the paper</u>   <u>Answer</u>

<u>ride</u> (present tense)   <u>rode</u> (past tense), r-o-d-e

come	do	eat	find	go
think	see	have	say	know
give	tell	get	hear	try
study	speak	swim	feel	spread
catch	put	shoot	cut	feed

Song
(group activity)

Learn the words and music to "That's What Friends Are For." This song was put together by a number of entertainers concerned about the spread of AIDS and in support of AIDS victims.

Small Group Discussions

In small groups, discuss the following controversial issues:

1. Should health care workers be required to submit to AIDS testing?
2. Should the law require AIDS victims to declare publicly that they carry the HIV virus?
3. Should the public school dispense condoms to students?
4. What more could be done to educate the public about the dangers of AIDS?

Unit 4

WOMEN'S
HEALTH

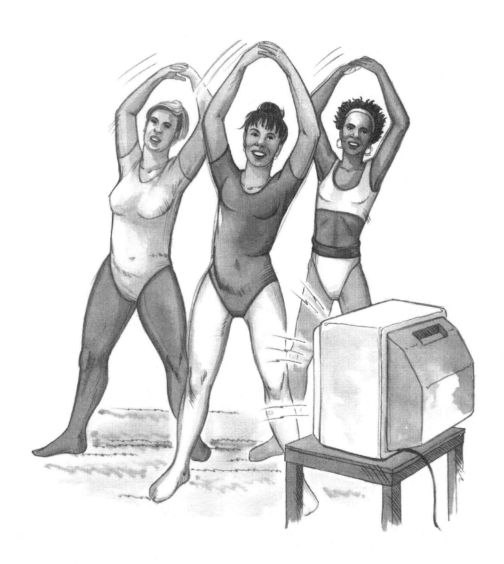

Annual Examination

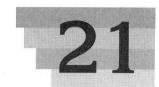

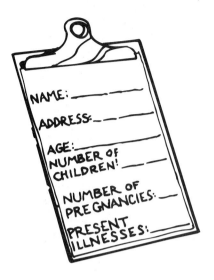

WORD LIST

Things
present
birth control
methods
menstrual period
cramp
breast exam
pelvic exam
news
pap smear
cervical cancer
breast cancer
mammogram

Actions
kiss
detect

Descriptions
personal

Next month is Theresa's birthday. Every year near her birthday, she has a physical exam. She knows that, like children, adults need physicals too.

This year Theresa is going in for her exam a month early because she isn't feeling well. She arrives at the doctor's office a little early because she knows she has to fill out forms.

Next Theresa goes into the examination room and changes into a gown. When the doctor comes in, Theresa explains that she feels tired all the time and sometimes her stomach is upset. The doctor begins by asking her questions, as follows, about her medical history:

1. How old are you?
2. How many times have you been pregnant?

3. How many children do you have?
4. Do you have any present illnesses?
5. Do you or does anyone in your family have a history of any illness such as tumors, cancer, heart disease, diabetes?
6. Do you smoke?
7. Have you ever smoked?
8. What kind of birth control do you use?
9. What birth control methods have you used?
10. When was your last menstrual period?
11. How often are your menstrual periods?
12. Do you have pain or cramps with periods?
13. Have you been in the hospital in the last five years?
14. Have you had any surgeries?

The doctor completes the physical by doing a breast exam and a pelvic exam. Theresa thinks doctors who do pelvic exams should be women.

The doctor says he'll call her with the test results only if there's a problem. He also suggests that she get a mammogram

But when Theresa's phone rings two days later, the doctor says "I have an early birthday present for you. You're going to have a baby!"

At first Theresa can't believe it. Then she tells Tomas and he can't believe it. Everything has been so busy since their move, they stopped thinking about a baby. But now they're hugging and kissing. They're so happy about the news!

Comprehension Check

Circle the correct answer.

1. What does Theresa do every year near her birthday?

   a. takes her children to the doctor   b. has a physical exam

   c. has a party

2. Why does Theresa go for her exam a month early?

   a. because she's feeling tired   b. because the doctor wants to see her

   c. because she knows adults need physicals too

3. When the doctor asks Theresa about her medical history, he asks questions about her family too.

    a. true   b. false

4. What doesn't the doctor give Theresa after he completes the physical?

    a. a breast exam   b. a pelvic exam   c. a lollipop

5. How does Theresa feel about the doctor's "birthday present"?

    a. happy   b. unhappy   c. worried

 Cultural Note

Some women are uncomfortable with all the questions that the doctor asks. They may not understand why she needs all the information she asks for. The questions may seem personal or difficult to answer. But a good doctor knows that health care is not a simple matter. She needs to know a lot about a patient to give the right help. A patient can help the doctor by giving as much information as the doctor wants.

Most women also find a pelvic exam uncomfortable. But a pap smear is part of a pelvic exam and it is the best way to detect cervical cancer. All women should have a pap smear at least once a year.

A breast exam is the easiest way to detect breast cancer. Once you know how, you can do it yourself once a month. Regular mammograms are also recommended for women 35 and over (see Lesson 22).

Word Search

Circle the following words in the puzzle. Words are across and down.

PERSONAL   ANNUAL   BIRTH CONTROL   SURGERY

PAP SMEAR   MEDICAL HISTORY   METHODS   BREAST EXAM

DETECT   PELVIC EXAM   MENSTRUAL PERIOD   HUGGING

CERVICAL CANCER   KISSING   CRAMP   PRESENT

```
M E N S T R U A L P E R I O D S I A
E T C I J R N I O R W V R H E A N N
D W Y H I W A L B E O E T R B W S N
I N A E N L V E H S U R G E R Y A U
C R A M P Y E R F E I S B K O Y E A
A E J L E B O T I N R F E L R S B L
L F I H L D B D E T E C T C A I A E
H C L E V K A C L M N A L Q K I J B
I L N J I L K M P E O N Q P C R N I
S L S S C E R V I C A L C A N C E R
T F P T E D U V F N W X P C F N T
O L E Y X B A M Z A B H Z S A Z J H
R A R I A K L E B M C U D M K M E C
Y F S G M B A M H J I G F E Z E L O
D F O H F K I S S I N G B A L T J N
M J N A K C L I L M N I H R D H D T
A O A I L D B M P U Z N A C N O B R
J K L Q T W Y H J I K G V C F D E O
S C R I B M X M O N R E B E E S G L
B R E A S T E X A M K H N D K L H H
```

Matching

Match the word with the meaning.

1. _____ touch with the lips
2. _____ a gift
3. _____ a recent event or events
4. _____ to find out
5. _____ private
6. _____ used to prevent pregnancy
7. _____ a sharp muscle pain
8. _____ ways of doing things

a. news
b. detect
c. personal
d. birth control
e. present
f. kiss
g. methods
h. cramp

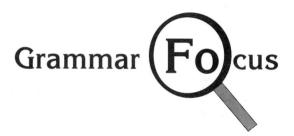

Grammar Focus

Questions using "what" and "how"

Questions asking for specific information about a thing (a noun) often begin with "what."

For example: <u>What</u> time is it?

Questions asking about the manner of something (an adverb) often begin with "how".

For example: <u>How</u> often do you do a breast exam?

Fill in the blanks below with "what" or "how."

1. _____ time is your appointment?
2. _____ hospital are you going to?
3. _____ was your visit to the doctor?
4. _____ often are your menstrual periods?

Write the number of the sentence above that fits each answer below.

5. _____ It was O.K.
6. _____ It's at 4:00.

7. _____ They're about every 28 days.

8. _____ I'm going to the county hospital.

Complete the following sentences with "what" or "how." Then write an answer.

9. Q: _____ many children do you have?

A: I _____

10. Q: _____ do you do on weekends?

A: I _____

What about you?

○ Do you think doctors ask questions that are too personal?

○ Do you have an annual examination every year? If not, why not?

══════ PRACTICE EXERCISES ══════

Cloze exercise: Past Tense
(individual or pair activity)

The first parapgraph below is written in the present tense. The second will be in the past tense as soon as you fill in the same verbs in the past tense. Some of the verbs are regular, and some are irregular.

Present Tense

Today Theresa (1) <u>has</u> an appointment for a physical examination. This time she (2) <u>is</u> going a month early because she (3) <u>isn't</u> feeling well. She (4) <u>arrives</u> at the doctor's office early because she (5) <u>knows</u> that she (6) <u>has</u> to fill out forms. Theresa (7) <u>goes</u> into an examination room and (8) <u>changes</u> into a gown. Then the doctor (9) <u>comes</u> in and (10) <u>examines</u> her. He (11) <u>begins</u> by asking her a lot of questions. Then he (12) <u>gives</u> her the physical exam. After the exam he (13) <u>tells</u> Theresa he will call her if he (14) <u>thinks</u> there (15) <u>is</u> anything she should know.

Past Tense

Last week Theresa (1) _____ an appointment for a physical examination. This time she (2) _____ going a month early because she (3) _____ feeling well. She (4) _____ the doctor's office early because she (5) _____ that she (6) _____ to fill out forms. Theresa (7) _____ into an examination room and (8) _____ into a gown. Then the doctor (9) _____ in and (10) _____ her. He (11) _____ by asking her a lot of questions. Then he (12) _____her the physical exam. After the exam he (13) _____ Theresa he will call her if he (14) _____ there (15) _____ anything she should know.

Formulating Questions
(pair activity)

This exercise is designed to help you put words in the correct order for questions. When your partner asks a question, do not answer it until the question is phrased correctly. You will have the correct phrasing on your page when you are the listener. Listen carefully. You may help your partner phrase it correctly, but do not answer the question until your partner says the question correctly. Partner B's section is in Appendix A, pages 230-231.

PARTNER A

1. Ask your partner if he/she has any children.
   Your partner's answer: _____
2. Listen and answer (when the question is phrased correctly):
   "Do you have any present illnesses?"
3. Ask your partner if he/she has ever smoked.
   Your partner's answer: _____
4. Listen and answer (when the question is phrased correctly):
   "When was your last physical examination?"

5. Ask your partner if he/she has been in the hospital in the last five years.
   Your partner's answer:_____

6. Listen and answer (when the question is phrased correctly)
   "When do you think they will find a cure for Aids?"

7. Ask your partner how he got to this class.
   Your partner's answer:_____

8. Listen and answer (when the question is phrased correctly)
   "Why did you take this class?"

9. Ask you partner why he/she doesn't like to go to the doctor.
   Your partner's answer:_____

10. Listen and answer (when the question is phrased correctly)
    "Would you like to lend me fifty dollars?"

Role Play

(group activity)

Act out the following situations (in groups of 3, 4, or 5). Be sure that everyone has something to say.

1. A mother keeps putting off her annual examination, even though *her* mother died of breast cancer two years ago. The rest of the family wants her to go get checked out by the doctor, but she keeps coming up with excuses on why she can't go. How does the rest of the family convince her to go?

2. A doctor is telling a husband and wife that the wife is pregnant (he has already examined her). The husband and wife are happy. Then the doctor tells them the big surprise: they are not going to have just one baby; They are going to have quintuplets (5) ! How do the husband and wife react?

3. A teenager (not married) must tell her parents that she thinks she is pregnant. She doesn't know for sure yet. How do the parents handle this?

4. Two women have come to the doctor's office at the same time, and they both want to be seen by the doctor immediately. One wants to know if she's pregnant (because she wants to be) and the other one wants to know if she's not pregnant (because she doesn't want to be). How does the receptionist handle these two anxious women?

5. A man is waiting for the doctor to come into the examination room. He has already changed into a gown. He gets bored waiting for the doctor so he starts talking to himself and absentmindedly playing with the switches on the wall. The doctor (outside the door) is late because he is being interviewed by a TV news reporter about some new medical discovery. By accident the man in the waiting room pulls the fire alarm. When he opens the door to try to explain what happened, there is the TV camera taking pictures of him in his skimpy gown. How does he try to show the doctor what happened and cover himself up for the camera at the same time?

6. A woman is in the examination room for her annual exam. The nurse asks her how old she is, how many times she has been pregnant, how many children she has, if she has any present illnesses, if anyone in her family has a history of any illnesses such as tumors, cancer, heart disease, or diabetes. The woman answers all these questions as the nurse marks off answers on a chart. Then the doctor comes in and introduces himself/herself. The doctor asks her if she smokes, if she has been in the hospital in the last five years, and if she has had any surgeries. Then the doctor gets called away on an emergency, and the woman has to reschedule her appointment.

22 Breast Examination

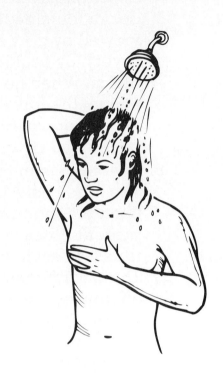

WORD LIST

Things
self-examination
lump
depression
nipple
decoloration
clockwise motion
mammogram

Actions
detect
promise
press
squeeze
treat
discharge

Descriptions
slippery
curable

When Theresa went for her physical examination, the doctor showed her how to do a breast self-examination to detect cancer, and she promised she would do it every month one week after her menstrual period. Theresa is much happier doing a self-examination than having the doctor do it.

First Theresa stands in front of the mirror and looks at each breast to see if there is a lump, a depression, or anything unusual about her breasts or nipples. Then she raises both arms over her head and looks for any swelling or depression of the skin, or discoloration of the nipples.

When Theresa gets in the shower and her skin is wet and slippery with soap, she raises her right arm over her head and with her left hand, using a clockwise motion, feels the right breast for a lump or anything unusual. Then she raises her left arm and repeats the motion.

After her shower, Theresa lies down and puts her right arm under her head and a small pillow under her right shoulder. Then she presses on the right breast, using a clockwise motion, and examines all parts of the breast. Next she squeezes the nipple to see if any discharge comes out. She repeats the motions for the left breast.

Theresa is glad she can do something to take care of her own health.

Comprehension Check

Circle the correct answer.

1. Theresa is glad she can do her own breast examination.

   a. true   b. false

2. What isn't Theresa looking for when she does a breast self-examination?

   a. a lump   b. a depression   c. a clock

3. How often does Theresa do a self-examination?

   a. once a year   b. once a month   c. twice a month

4. When does Theresa do a self-examination?

   a. one week after her period   b. one week before her period

   c. on the first day of each month

5. Why does Theresa do a breast self-examination?

   a. to feel her pulse   b. to detect cancer   c. to check her breathing

More Information

Breast cancer usually occurs in women in their forties and fifties and is the most common cancer among women. In fact, one in every 11 women gets breast cancer. But if it is detected and treated early, it is usually curable. If it is treated late, it is much more dangerous.

So a breast self-exam every month is very important. It could save your life. Of course most lumps in your breast (3 out of 4) are not cancerous, but you should tell a doctor right away if you find anything unusual. Tell a doctor even if you're worried or you have no money. It could save your life.

Regular mammograms are also recommended as follows:
- ○ age 35 to 39   first mammogram
- ○ age 40 to 49   every 1 to 2 years
- ○ age 50+   every year

Fill in the Blank

Fill in the blanks with the correct word from the list below.

lump	nipples
clockwise	menstrual period
depression	discharge
squeeze	self-examination

Every woman should do a breast (1) _____ every month one week after her (2) _____ _____ . Look for any (3)_____ or (4) _____ on the breasts or on the (5) _____. Next, raise one arm at a time over your head and feel each breast with a (6) _____ motion. Then lie down and (7) _____ each nipple to check for (8) _____.

Word Groups

Put each word from the list below in the correct group.

nipple	press	breast
swelling	discharge	squeeze
depression	clockwise motion	self-examination
lump		

What to do:

_____

Where to look:

_____

_____

Things to look for:

_____

_____

_____

How to look:

_____

_____

Grammar 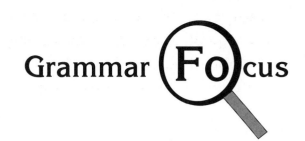cus

Comparatives

Form the comparative by adding "er" to a description word. The description word is usually followed by "than".

> *For example:* Flying is safer than driving.

When the description word has three or more syllables, use "more" in place of "er".

> *For example:* Mark is more impatient than Cathy.

Fill in the blanks with the correct words.

> *For example:* The red book is (large) _____ the blue book.
> The red book is <u>larger</u> <u>than</u> the blue book.

1. Treating breast cancer late is much (dangerous) _____ treating it early.

2. Thomas is (tall) _____ Theresa.

3. Theresa is (happy) _____ doing a breastself-examination _____ having the doctor do it.

   (*Note:* In this sentence, "than" is separated from the comparative.)

4. Winter is (cold) _____ fall.

5. Cathy is (quiet) _____ her brother.

6. She is (beautiful) _____ any woman I have ever seen.

7. Children are usually (noisy)_____ adults.

8. I think reading is (interesting)_____ watching television.

What about you?

○ What are the four steps of a breast self-exam?
1.
2.
3.
4.

○ Do you know how to do a breast self-exam?

○ Do you do your own breast self-exam? If so, how often?

PRACTICE EXERCISES

Comparatives and Superlatives
(small group activity)

In your group, compose 5 questions to ask the rest of the class. In your questions you may use anyone or anything in the classroom, but use the *comparative* or *superlative* forms of 5 of the following adjectives:

Adjective	Comparative	Superlative
tall	taller	tallest
big	bigger	biggest
exciting	more exciting	most exciting
interesting	more interesting	most interesting
small	smaller	smallest
funny	funnier	funniest
heavy	heavier	heaviest
short	shorter	shortest
good	better	best
bad	worse	worst
embarassing	more embarassing	most embarassing
comfortable	more comfortable	most comfortable
easy	easier	easiest
difficult	more difficult	most difficult

Examples: 1. Who is taller, Gloria or David?
2. Who tells the funniest jokes in the class?
3. Which is heavier, the teacher's desk or your desk?

4. Which language is easier to learn, English or Spanish?

5. Who has a more difficult job, the teacher or the students?

Questions:

1._____?

2._____?

3._____?

4._____?

5._____?

Conversation
(pair activity)

With a partner, read or respond to the following. Then change roles and repeat the process. Be sure that your partner makes the correct choice.

PARTNER A

1. Theresa went to the doctor. A month later she had a birthday.
2. Theresa does a self-examination of her breasts every month. She does not want to miss the early signs of breast cancer.
3. Breast cancer is the most common cancer in women, but it is curable if it is detected early.
4. Theresa sat in the doctor's waiting room for 15 minutes. Then the nurse called her into the examination room.
5. If Theresa does not do this self-examination every month, she may miss the early signs of breast cancer.
6. The doctor examined Theresa. Then he told her to get a mammogram.
7. During the examination the doctor was telling Theresa how to give herself an examination every month.

PARTNER B

1. a. Theresa had a birthday <u>after</u> she went to the doctor.
   b. Theresa had a birthday <u>before</u> she went to the doctor.

2. a. Theresa examines herself <u>unless</u> she doesn't want to miss the early signs of cancer.

  b. Theresa examines herself <u>because</u> she doesn't want to miss the early signs of cancer.

3. a. <u>Until</u> breast cancer is the most common cancer in women, it is not dangerous if detected early.

  b. <u>Although</u> breast cancer is the most common cancer in women, it is not dangerous if detected early.

4. a. Theresa sat in the waiting room <u>although</u> the nurse called her name.

  b. Theresa sat in the waiting room <u>until</u> the nurse called her name.

5. a. <u>Unless</u> Theresa examines herself every month, she will miss the early signs of cancer.

  b. <u>Because</u> Theresa examines herself every month, she will miss the early signs of cancer.

6. a. The doctor examined Theresa <u>after</u> he told her to get a mammogram.

  b. The doctor examined Theresa <u>before</u> he told her to get a mammogram.

7. a. The doctor was talking to Theresa <u>while</u> he was examining her.

  b. The doctor was talking to Theresa <u>although</u> he was examining her.

Reflexive Pronouns
(pair activity)

Study the following list of reflexive pronouns:

Singular	Plural
myself	ourselves
yourself	yourselves
himself	themselves
herself	
itself	

Working with a partner, fill in the blanks in the following chart. Be sure to use the correct reflexive pronoun. *Do not look at your partner's chart* during the exercise, but compare your answers afterwards to make sure you both did it correctly. Partner B's chart is in Appendix A, pages 231-232.

PARTNER A

Ask your partner, "What did _____ do?"

Person	Activity	Reflexive Pronoun	Rest of Sentence
Theresa	_____	herself	a day off.
Thomas	cut	_____	shaving.
We	congratulated	_____	on our good grades.
They	_____	themselves	on television.
The dog	scratched	_____	behind its ear.
You	_____	yourself	one of the family.
You two	hurt	_____	on the ice.
I	_____	myself	a present.
Ana and Ed	saw	_____	in the wall mirror.
He	_____	himself	for the struggle ahead.

23   Prenatal Care

WORD LIST

Things

Brussels sprouts
rice

pork chops
fruit salad
protein
calories
calcium
problems
nurse practitioner
heartbeat
capsule
product
substitute
well-being

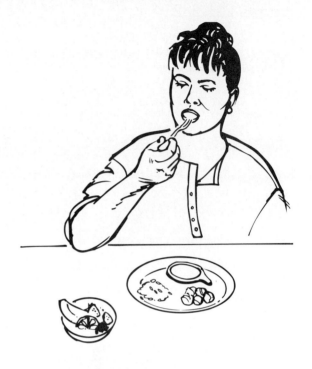

Actions

assure

Descriptions

prenatal
fetal
well-balanced

"Let's see, Brussel sprouts, rice, pork chops, fruit salad . . ." Theresa is thinking about what to make for dinner. Cathy and Mark don't like Brussel sprouts at all, but now that Theresa's pregnant, she has to think carefully about her diet. Her doctor told her that she must eat 50% more protein and about 300 calories more per day. Also, at least once a day, Theresa drinks nonfat milk and eats milk products for the calcium.

It's a good thing Tomas stopped smoking, because babies born to mothers who breathe smoke can have a lower birth weight and other health problems. And Theresa is not going to drink any alcohol, not even a glass of wine with dinner, because she read that the alcohol will pass into the baby's blood. Even any medication that Theresa takes will affect the baby.

Theresa is going to continue with her walking for exercise too, although she gets tired more quickly now. Often Cathy walks with her, and sometimes they talk about the baby. Cathy wants to know if she will still have her own room when they have another child around. Theresa is glad Cathy walks with her and they talk together.

Theresa feels good, too. Being pregnant gives her a sense of well-being. The only problem is finding time to visit the doctor. For the first 28 weeks of pregnancy, Theresa has been visiting the doctor once a month, but soon she is going to start going every two weeks. Life is busy for a working mother! Maybe Tomas will cook the Brussels sprouts tonight.

Comprehension Check

Circle the correct answer.

1. What is the Santos family having for dinner tonight?

   a. Brussel sprouts, potatoes, and pork chops

   b. rice, Brussel sprouts, and pork chops   c. pork chops, peas, and rice

2. Theresa must eat less during her pregnancy.

   a. true   b. false

3. Theresa must eat 50% more _____ during pregnancy.

   a. protein   b. rice   c. vegetables

4. Why does Theresa drink milk?

   a. to gain weight   b. to lose weight   c. for the calcium

5. What doesn't Theresa drink during her pregnancy?

   a. alcohol   b. milk   c. tea

6. What does Theresa have to think carefully about during pregnancy?

   a. diet   b. breast exam   c. smoking

More Information

The purpose of prenatal care is to help assure the birth of a healthy baby. During pregnancy the most important thing for a mother to remember is that everything she does will now affect two people, not just one.

But a doctor or nurse practitioner is there to help. After the first physical examination, the pregnant woman makes an appointment once a month for the first 28 weeks, then every two weeks until 36 weeks, then once a week. It is important that a doctor check blood pressure, weight, urine, fetal heartbeat, and fetal growth at these appointments.

Total weight gain should be 24 to 27 pounds and there should be no weight loss at any time during pregnancy.

Nutrition, of course, is very important. Often the doctor will prescribe vitamin and mineral capsules in addition to a well-balanced diet. The following is a recommended eating plan for pregnant women and women who are breast-feeding:

Suggested Daily Food Group Servings at 3 Calorie Levels for Women who are Pregnant or Breastfeeding	Not Active 1,600 calories	Moderately Active 2,200 calories	Very Active 2,800 calories
Bread group servings	6	9	11
Vegetable group servings	3	4	5
Fruit group servings	2	3	4
Milk group servings	3	3	3
Meat group servings	5	6	7
Total fat (grams)	53	73	93
Total added sugars (teaspoons)	6	12	18

Crossword Puzzle

Fill in the words from the word list below.

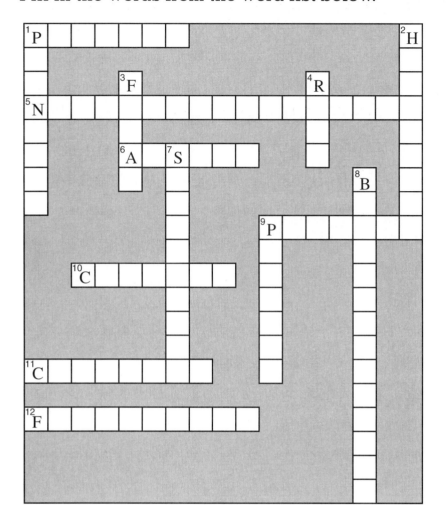

fetal
calcium
rice
protein
prenatal
Brussels
  sprout
substitute
heartbeat
problem
nurse practi-
tioner
calories
assure
fruit salad
product

ACROSS

1. eggs and fish are a good source for this
5. sometimes this person will see you instead of the doctor
6. to make sure of something
9. cheese is a type of milk
   _____
10. milk is a good source for this
11. Theresa needs to increase her _____ by 300 a day
12. apples, pears, grapes mixed together

DOWN

1. mothers need this care before the baby is born
2. what the doctor hears when he listens to your chest
3. unborn or still in the womb
4. a white grain
7. to replace one thing for another
8. a small vegetable that looks like a cabbage
9. a difficult situation

Grammar 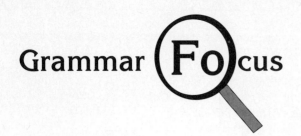cus

Future tense using "going to"

Use the future tense to express an action that is going to happen in the future. Form the future tense by using the appropriate form of the verb "to be" + "going to" before the infinitive form of the verb.

For example: Theresa <u>is going to have</u> a baby.

Change the following sentences to the future tense.

1. Theresa drinks nonfat milk for the calcium.

   _____.

2. Tomas stopped smoking.

   _____.

3. Theresa continues with her walking for exercise.

   _____.

4. Cathy walks with her mother.

   _____.

Write two sentences from the story that tell what Theresa is going to do while she's pregnant.

5. _____.

6. _____.

Write two sentences that tell things you're going to do in the next week.

7. _____.

8. _____.

Think About This

1. What are some foods that are high in calcium?

2. What are some foods that are high in protein?

3. Name some milk products.

4. Name some meat substitutes.

5. What are some dark green or yellow vegetables?

6. What are some citrus fruits?

══════ PRACTICE EXERCISES ══════

Vocabulary Match-Up

Your teacher will give you a slip of paper with one of the following
items. Find the person whose slip matches the word or definition on
your slip of paper. Stay with your partner until the class rules it a correct
match.

prenatal care	○ part of the bread food group
capsule	○ normal weight gain in pregnancy
citrus fruits	
vegetables	○ to give confidence to; to make sure
meat, eggs, poultry	
milk products	○ checkups and any necessary medical attention before birth
fetal	
rice	○ lemons, limes, grapefruits, oranges
alcoholic drinks	
24-27 pounds	○ a certain type of pill
well-being	○ something that can harm the fetus during pregnancy
assure	
	○ good sources of calcium
	○ good health
	○ spinach, Brussels sprouts, peas, carrots
	○ unborn, still in the womb
	○ good sources of protein

Small Group Activity

In groups of 4 or 5, plan a healthy breakfast, lunch, dinner, and snack for Theresa. Be sure to select foods from each of the major food groups for a balanced diet. Remember that her doctor said that she must eat 50% more protein and about 300 more calories per day (don't make them "empty calories"!). Present your diet to the class, and be prepared to justify your choices.

Find Someone in the Class Who . . .

1. knows someone who is pregnant _____
2. is a victim of secondary smoke at home _____
3. hates Brussels sprouts _____
4. eats a well-balanced diet every day _____
5. never drinks milk _____
6. is on a special diet _____
7. has never had an alcoholic drink _____
8. exercises by walking at least 3 times a week _____
9. never seems to have enough time for anything _____
10. never wants to get pregnant _____

Breast-Feeding

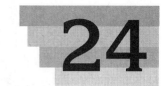

24

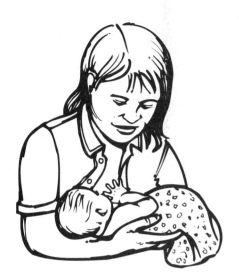

WORD LIST

<u>Things</u>
breast-feeding
antibody
infection
breast pump
liquid
uterus

<u>Actions</u>
suck

<u>Descriptions</u>
allergic
daily
normal
emotionally

Theresa's baby is due in about a month. She's thinking about breast-feeding. She breast-fed her other children, but that was a long time ago. Now only about half of all babies are breast-fed, probably because so many mothers are working. Theresa herself wasn't working when Mark and Cathy were babies.

Theresa thinks breast-feeding is a good idea, for the following reasons:

○ A mother's milk has the right nutrition.
○ It's easy to digest.
○ It gives the baby antibodies to protect against diseases and infections.
○ Babies are usually not allergic to breast milk.
○ It's always clean, fresh, and at the right temperature.
○ It's there when the baby needs it.

The difficulty with breast feeding is that no one but the mother can do it. But Theresa's neighbor Ana told her about a breast pump that mothers can use to save their milk in bottles. Theresa likes that idea since she's planning to go back to work part-time about eight weeks after the baby is born. She's also glad that Ana promised to help with the baby and help her learn to breast-feed again. It's been a long time! What a lot of things to think about!

Comprehension Check

Circle the correct answer.

1. Of all babies, about how many are breast-fed?

    a. only a few   b. about half   c. almost all

2. Breast milk is the most nutritious kind of milk.

    a. true   b. false

3. Antibodies protect against _____.

    a. infections   b. allergies   c. digestion

4. Breast milk isn't _____.

    a. too warm   b. fresh   c. clean

5. What is the most difficult thing about breast-feeding?

    a. babies don't like it   b. only the mother can do it

    c. it's not good for babies

6. What does Theresa do to prepare for breast-feeding?

    a. uses a breast pump   b. goes back to work

    c. asks Ana to show her how to breast-feed

More Information

To have enough milk for their babies, mothers must eat a good diet. (See "Daily Food Guide for Women" in Lesson 23—Prenatal Care). Breast-feeding mothers should also drink 8 to 12 glasses of liquid daily. They should stay away from alcohol, however.

But with all of these "shoulds" for the baby, a breast-feeding mother should understand she's also helping herself. Breast-feeding makes her uterus return to normal size more quickly after pregnancy. And it helps her lose the weight she gained during pregnancy. Breast milk costs nothing, and when the baby sucks it brings mother and child close emotionally.

Some women, however, feel they should breast-feed only when they are at home and when they are alone with their baby. Finding this time may be difficult for them. Also, any mother who must take medication should ask a doctor about breast-feeding because many medications can be passed to the baby in breast milk.

Fill in the Blank

Fill in the blanks with the correct words from the list below:

infection   breast-feeding
sucks   emotionally
antibodies   breast pump
nutrition   uterus
daily   allergic

Eating well is always important, but good (1) _____

is especially important when a mother is (2) _____.

Mother and baby both need vitamins and minerals (3) _____.

Breast milk has (4) _____ to protect a baby from

(5) _____ which will make her sick.

Breast milk is easy to digest and babies are usually not

(6) _____ to it.

If a mother cannot be with her baby at all feeding times, she can

use a (7) _____ _____ and put breast

milk in bottles.

If a mother has a baby who (8) _____ breast milk,

her (9) _____ will return to normal size more

quickly. Also, she and her baby will be close (10) _____.

Grammar 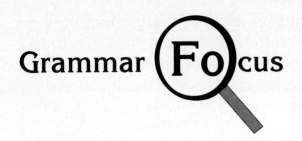 cus

Past Tense

Use the past tense to express an action that happened in the past. Form the past tense of regular verbs by adding "ed" to the infinitive form of the verb.

> *For example:* Tomas <u>stopped</u> smoking.
>
> (*Note:* When the final consonant of the verb is preceded by a vowel, double the final consonant before adding "ed".)
> Irregular verbs have special past tense forms.

> *For example:* Theresa <u>began</u> drinking more milk before the baby was born.

Write the following sentences in the past tense.

1. Theresa likes using a breast pump.

_____.

2. He walks to work.

_____.

3. She breast-feeds her baby.

_____.

4. Theresa learns to breast-feed from Ana.

_____.

Write two sentences from the story that tell about something that happened in the past.

5. _____.

6. _____.

Write two sentences about things *you* did in the past week.

7. _____.

8. _____.

PRACTICE EXERCISES

Advantage or Disadvantage?
(pair activity)

On a piece of paper make two columns, one labeled "Advantages" and the other "Disadvantages." Discuss the following with a partner, and put each one under one or the other category. Feel free to add more of your own.

Breast-Feeding

- In the middle of the night, the father cannot get up and feed the baby.
- Breast milk is easy to digest.
- Babies are usually not allergic to breast milk.
- A breast-feeding-mother's breasts are larger than normal.
- A breast-feeding mother should not drink alcoholic beverages.
- Breast milk is always at the right temperature.
- A working mother must use a breast pump and plan ahead a lot.
- A mother's milk has the right nutrition.
- Breast-feeding mothers sometimes get stains on their blouses.
- Breast milk gives babies antibodies.
- It is sometimes not easy to breast-feed a baby in a public place.

After you have finished, be ready to tell the class whether you think it is better to breast-feed or bottle-feed a baby.

Small Group Discussions

Some women have been asked to leave restaurants or other public places because they were breast-feeding their babies. Discuss when and where you think it is appropriate for a mother to breast-feed her baby. Be prepared to present your conclusions to the class.

Pronunciation Exercise

(pair activity)

Copy the following lists of words (Partner A's are listed here. Partner B's are in Appendix A, pages 233-234.) Where it says "Listen and check" put a check mark by the word your partner pronounces. Where it says "Pronounce" say the word that is underlined, and your partner will put a check mark by that word. *Do not look at your partner's page.* When you are finished, correct your answers. If you don't know how to pronounce a word, ask the teacher.

PARTNER A

1. Listen and check:

risk	_____
disk	_____
list	_____

2. Pronounce:

shared

sheared

<u>share</u>

3. Listen and check:

flight	_____
fright	_____
fight	_____

4. Pronounce:

cute

<u>quit</u>

quite

5. Listen and check:

law	_____
low	_____
raw	_____

6. Pronounce:

<u>bland</u>

blend

plan

7. Listen and check:

been	_____
bean	_____
bane	_____

8. Pronounce:

police

<u>policy</u>

bodice

9. Listen and check:

proud	_____
plowed	_____
prude	_____

10. Pronounce:

<u>expansive</u>

especially

expensive

11. Pronounce:

seen

sighed

<u>sign</u>

12. Listen and check:

berry   _____

very   _____

belly   _____

13. Pronounce:

eyes

AIDS

<u>ides</u>

14. Listen and check:

busy   _____

visa   _____

visit   _____

Choral Reading: Song

(group activity)

For many pregnant women the final month seems like a year. Sing the following song to the tune of "I've Been Working on the Railroad." Pay attention to the rhythm of the words. This will help your pronunciation and intonation.

Theresa's Song

I've been waiting for this baby
All the whole year long
I've been waiting for this baby
Doctor, is the due date wrong?
Can't my labor start tomorrow
There's a pain, I could have sworn!
Wake me up when it's all over
Tell me that it's born.

Baby, don't you know?
Baby, don't you know?
Baby. don't you know you're due?
Baby, don't you know?
Baby, don't you know?
What your mama's going through?

Someone told my baby the wrong date
Someone told my baby, I know
Someone told my baby the wrong date
When he was an embryo.

(Alternate ending: "That's why he is oh, so slow.")

Dice Game
(group activity)

Taking turns, move the number of spaces you roll on the die. If you land on an empty square, stay there and wait for your next turn. If you land on a square with a sentence, say whether it is correct or incorrect. If it is incorrect, correct it. If you are right, move ahead two squares. If you are incorrect, move back two squares.

FINISH 50	90% of all babies are now breast-fed. 49	Most babies are allergic to breast milk. 48	47	Medication can be passed to the baby through breast milk. 46
41	"Prenatal" means "after the baby is born." 42	43	Milk is a good source of calcium. 44	45
"Rice" rhymes with "police." 40	39	Secondary smoke can affect unborn babies. 38	37	Apples are citrus fruits. 36
31	A woman should gain 40 to 50 lbs. during pregnancy. .32	33	34	"Breast" rhymes with "guest." 35
"This book is more better" is correct English. 30	29	28	A breast self-exam should be done every month. 27	26
21	22	The most common cancer in women is lung cancer. 23	24	Pap smears help to detect cervical cancer. 25
20	"Gown" rhymes with "grown." 19	18	"Annual" means "every month." 17	16
Today he gives; yesterday he gaves. 11	12	"Why you took this class?" is correct English. 13	14	You can get AIDS by sharing a drug needle. 15
10	"Missed" is pronounced just like "mist." 9	You can get AIDS by hugging an AIDS victim. 8	7	"Sign" rhymes with "mine." 6
START	"Rehabilitation" means "becoming addicted." 2	3	A mammogram helps find breast cancer in women. 4	An addict is a person who never uses drugs. 5

Baby Care

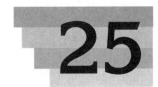

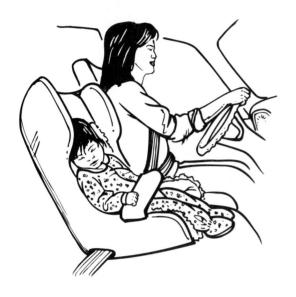

Things
crib
kitten
diaper
car seat
law
rash
object
button

Actions
due
plan
roll over
pick up
support
wake up

Descriptions
padded
public
soiled
mild
careful
unattended
fragile

Nothing is going right these days at the Santos' house. Everyone is thinking about the baby that's due any day. This morning Tomas was late for work because Ana brought over a crib and he couldn't decide where the baby would sleep most comfortably. This afternoon Cathy brought a kitten home from school and told her mother it was for the baby. Yesterday Theresa brought 72 diapers home, and then couldn't find them. Mark thinks everyone is completely crazy, especially because today he found the 72 diapers in his room!

Well, it's good Theresa is trying to plan for the baby. She's glad Ana brought over a crib with padded sides so the baby won't get hurt. Theresa also got a car seat for the baby from Ana. The law requires that all children up to 40 pounds must ride in a special car seat. The doctor, however, told Theresa not to take the baby out to public places or around a lot of people for at least two weeks.

Theresa also talked with the doctor about skin care. She remembers from her other two children that wet or soiled diapers can cause diaper rash. That's why she bought 72 diapers and will clean the baby carefully after each diaper change. And the doctor reminded her to use a mild soap to give the baby a bath every day. Theresa remembers how Tomas used to give Mark and Cathy baths when they were little. They had a good time together. With Tomas's help, having a baby around is a lot easier!

Four days later Theresa had a healthy baby boy weighing seven pounds eight ounces. Congratulations Tomas and Theresa on your new son, Samuel!

Comprehension Check

Circle the correct answer.

1. When is the baby due?

   a. in a month   b. any day   c. in a week

2. What did Theresa buy?

   a. 72 diapers   b. a kitten   c. a crib

3. What didn't Theresa get from Ana?

   a. a crib   b. a car seat   c. diapers

4. The crib has _____.

   a. a car seat   b. padded sides   c. padded legs

5. Children up to _____ pounds need a car seat.

   a. 40   b. 20   c. 60

6. What must Theresa do to prevent diaper rash?

   a. change the baby's diapers often   b. clean the baby carefully

   c. both a and b

More Information

Your baby's safety is the most important thing to think about. Don't leave him unattended where he can roll over, fall, or find small objects to put in his mouth. And don't leave him unattended with a bottle in case he starts choking.

Here are ten ways to make your home child-safe:

- ○ Cover unused outlets.
- ○ Keep thin plastic wrapping material away from children.
- ○ Keep small objects out of reach of children.
- ○ Remove free falling lids from storage containers.
- ○ Turn all handles of pots and pans towards the back of the stove.
- ○ Keep cleaning products and medicine above a child's reach.
- ○ Keep sharp objects above a child's reach.
- ○ Unplug appliances not in use.
- ○ Check extension cords for wear and don't use them if there is exposed wire.
- ○ Keep emergency and poison control center numbers handy.

Be sure your baby is on her back when you pick her up, and always support her head. Babies are not as fragile as we think, but they do need special care.

All babies have their own special needs. Some babies want to eat every two hours, some every four hours. Some babies sleep all night, some wake up every few hours. But all babies cry to let you know they want something. You'll learn the different ways your baby cries so you'll know what's wrong.

Do's and Dont's

Mark the correct answer.

	Do	Don't
1. let your baby lie down in the car		
2. listen to the way your baby cries		
3. pick up your baby when he's on his stomach		
4. let your baby sleep unattended on a bed		
5. cook dinner while your baby is drinking from a bottle		
6. let your baby have buttons to play with		
7. put your baby in a car seat when you take her in the car		
8. leave your baby on the sofa while you answer the phone in another room		
9. change your baby's diaper often		
10. give your baby a bath every day		
11. leave the iron on when you go in another room		
12. put your cleaning products on a low shelf		

Word Groups

Cross out the word that does *not* belong.

1. diaper   car seat   plan   crib

2. pick up   padded   wake up   roll over

3. object   kitten   button   unattended

4. wake up   padded   fragile   careful

Multiple Choice

Circle the correct answer.

1. Wet or soiled diapers can cause a diaper _____.

   rash   crib

2. If you don't pay attention to something it is _____.

   unattended   fragile

3. If children under forty pounds ride in a car they must

   be in a _____.

   diaper   car seat

4. Something which is easily hurt is _____.

   fragile   careful

5. Small red spots on the skin:

   rash   object

6. Another word that means "hold" is _____.

   plan   support

7. Ana brought over a crib with _____ sides.

   mild   padded

8. A word that means the opposite of "strong" is _____.

   mild   careful

9. What do you do in the morning before you get up?

   go to sleep   wake up

10. A word that means something is expected is _____.

    due   plan

Grammar 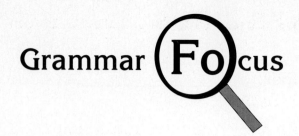cus

Past tense

Use the past tense to express an action that happened in the past. Irregular verbs have special past tense forms.

Use one of the following irregular past-tense forms to complete each of the following sentences. Words can be used more than once.

came	thought	was	had
read	gave	brought	told

1. Yesterday I _____ a bad cold.

2. This morning Tomas _____ late for work.

3. Ana _____ over a crib with padded sides.

4. I _____ the newspaper late last night.

5. Theresa _____ a healthy baby boy.

6. Mark _____ everyone _____ completely crazy.

7. She _____ to school with her brother.

8. The doctor _____ Theresa not to take the baby out in public at first.

9. This afternoon Cathy _____ a kitten home from school.

10. Tomas _____ Mark and Cathy baths when they were little.

PRACTICE EXERCISES

Art Project
(Individual or Pair Activity)

Draw a picture of the ideal nursery for a baby. You have unlimited funds, so you can have anything you want. When you have finished, write at least 10 sentences about what *would* be in your ideal nursery, and what the baby (or parent) *could do* there. Be sure to use the words *would* and *could*. (Remember that this is an imaginary nursery.) Please label everything in the nursery, also, so that the person who reads what you have written will know where to look on the picture.

Baby Shower
(group activity)

Your group of four or five students has been invited to a baby shower for the new mother. Decide what you will get for Theresa's new baby and report to the class.

Role Play
(group activity)

Act out the following situations (in groups of 3, 4, or 5). Be sure that everyone in the group has something to say.

1. A babysitter is trying to take care of four kids who keep doing dangerous things (you decide what). How does the babysitter cope?
2. The toys in the nursery are discussing how the children in the house use them and abuse them. Two of the toys are not safe (you decide why). What do they have to say to and about each other?
3. Everyone is very confused today. The delivery men are delivering the crib, and the mother can't decide where to put it. One child cannot find his clothes and keeps asking the mother where they are. A teenage child keeps talking on the phone. Suddenly the mother goes into labor. The teenager doesn't want to get off the phone, the delivery men just want the mother to sign a paper so they can get out of there, and the child starts to cry. How will this situation be resolved? (You may need a sixth person here.)

4. Three or four parents are watching their children play in the park. Each parent thinks that his/her child is the most coordinated, the most precocious (smart), the most advanced socially, and the best looking. How does each parent let the others know that his/her child is the superior one?

5. A 2 year-old baby has a very dirty diaper. His older brother, older sister, mother, and father all suddenly have something else to do. What excuses do they give for not being able to change the diaper? How do they decide who finally has to do it?

Bibliography

American Cancer Society. *Breast Self-Examination*. Atlanta: The American Cancer Society, 1988.

American Red Cross. *Aids and Children*. Washington D.C.: U.S. Public Health Service, 1986.

Ammer, Christine. The A to Z of Women's Health. New York: Everest House, 1983.

Baron, Jason D. *A Parent's Handbook of Drug Abuse Prevention and Treatment*. New York: The Putnam Publishing Group, 1983.

Gibb, Betty. Dental Health Adviser. *Your Child's First Visit*. Knoxville: Whittle Communications, 1988.

Hatch, Marilyn G. *Beyond Band-Aids and Kisses: First Aid Care for Children*. Spokane: Happy Home Publishing, 1986.

Health and Welfare Agency/Department of Health Services Immunization Unit. *Only IZs Will Protect Your Little One From . . .*Berkeley, CA 1991.

Krames Communication. *Preventing Hepatitis B for Health Care Workers*. Daly City, CA, 1989.

Kroeger, Robert F. Dental Health Adviser. *Conquer Dental Fear*. Knoxville: Whittle Communications, 1988.

Meyer, Roberta. *The Parent Connection: How to Communicate With Your Child About Alcohol and Other Drugs*. New York: Franklin Watts, 1984.

Norvell, Candyce. Dental Health Adviser. *A Cavity-Free Child*. Knoxville Whittle Communications,1988.

Pantell, Robert H., Fries, James F., and Vickery, Donald M. *Taking Care of Your Child*, revised edition. Reading: Addison-Wesley Publishing Co., 1984.

Reeder, Sharon J., Mastroianni, Luigi Jr., and Martin, Loenide, L. *Maternity Nursing*, 14th edition. Philadelphia: J.B. Lippincott Company, 1980.

Robinson, Corrine H. *Basic Nutrition and Diet Therapy*. New York: Macmillian Publishing Co. Inc., 1975.

San Mateo County AIDS Project. *AIDS*. San Mateo Department of Public Health, 1987.

U.S Department of Agriculture/Human Nutrition Information Services. *Food Guide Pyramid*. Hyattsville, MD, 1992.

U.S. Department of Health and Human Services/Public Health Service. National Institute on Alcohol Abuse and Alcholism. *Alcohol: Some Questions and Answers*. Washington, D.C.: U.S. Government Printing Office.

U.S. Department of Health and Human Services/Public Health Service. *Prenatal Care*. Rockville, MD, 1983.

Appendix A

Lesson 2: Oral Care: *Pronunciation Exercise*
(pair activity)

Copy the following lists of words for Partner B. (Partner A's list is on page 18.) Where it says "Listen and check" put a check mark by the word your partner pronounces. Where it says "Pronounce" say the word that is underlined, and your partner will put a check mark by that word. *Do not look at your partner's page.* When you are finished, correct your answers. If you don't know how to pronounce a word, ask the teacher.

PARTNER B

1. Pronounce:

   floss

   <u>flaws</u>

   flows

2. Listen and check:

   hum _____

   gum _____

   whom _____

3. Pronounce:

   tenth

   <u>teeth</u>

   tooth

4. Listen and check:

   done _____

   tong _____

   tongue _____

5. Listen and check:

   <u>black</u>

   plaque

   block

6. Listen and check:

   "h" (the letter) _____

   ace _____

   ache _____

7. Pronounce:

   <u>mouth</u>

   moth

   month

8. Listen and check:

   called _____

   cawed _____

   cold _____

9. Pronounce:		10. Listen and check:	
come		cute	_____
comb		caught	_____
calm		cut	_____
11. Pronounce:		**12.** Listen and check:	
racer		shore	_____
razor		sure	_____
resort		shower	_____

Lesson 4:   Exercise and Weight Control: *Information Gaps*
(pair activity; past tense, asking questions)

Ask your partner for the information for your blank boxes. Use the conversation below. Write the information in your boxes. *Do not look at your partner's page.*

PARTNER B

A: What did_____do yesterday at _____?
B: He/she_____. (Be sure to fill in the correct past tense)

Name	6:30 A. M.	4:30 P. M.	8:30 P. M.
Jim Nasium		(lift) _____ weights	(swim) _____ a mile
Ann Exercise	(ride) _____ a bike		
Dan D. Dancer		(play) _____ tennis	
C. Potato	(sleep) _____ through his alarm		(have) _____ a heart attack

Lesson 5: Taking Your Temperature: *Information Groups*

(pair activity; past tense, asking questions)

Ask your partner for the information for your blank boxes. Use the conversation below. Write the information in your boxes. *Do not look at your*

PARTNER B

A: What is _____'s temperature?

B: His/her temperature is _____ degrees.

A: What are his/her other symptoms?

B: He/she has _____.

Name	Temperature	Symptom	Symptom
Ann Teabody		a headache	
Mike Robe	102.8		a cough
Scarlet O'Fever			the chills
Rob Itussin	99.6	a runny nose	

Lesson 7: First Aid: *Pronunciation Exercise*
(pair activity)

Copy the following lists of words (Partner A's are on pages 58-59). Where it says "Listen and check" put a check mark by the word your partner pronounces. Where it says "Pronounce" say the word that is underlined, and your partner will put a check mark by that word. *Do not look at your partner's page.* When you are finished, correct your answers. If you don't know how to pronounce a word, ask the teacher.

PARTNER B

1. Pronounce:
   add
   aid
   I'd

2. Listen and check:
   put _____
   pat _____
   pet _____

3. Pronounce:
   laughed
   lift
   left

4. Listen and check:
   burn _____
   barn _____
   born _____

5. Pronounce:
   blaze
   blues
   bruise

6. Listen and check:
   heart _____
   girt _____
   hurt _____

7. Pronounce:
   perk
   park
   pork

8. Listen and check:
   sure _____
   sore _____
   sour _____

9. Pronounce:
   eyes
   ace
   ice

10. Listen and check:
    cold _____
    called _____
    sold _____

11. Pronounce:

<u>rungs</u>

wrens

runs

12. Listen and check:

water _____

wetter _____

waiter _____

13. Pronounce:

falls

feels

<u>fills</u>

14. Listen and check:

clan _____

cling _____

clean _____

Lesson 8: Emergency Services: *Giving Information to 911*

(pair activity)

Ask your partner for the information for your blank boxes. Use the conversation below. Write the information in your boxes. *Do not look at your partner's page*

PARTNER B

A: What is _____'s _____?

B: His _____ is _____.

Name	Phone No.	Problem	Address	Cross St.
Maria		baby choking		Park Ave.
Juan	474-5581			Tate Blvd.
Samuel		house on fire	10 Downing Dr.	

Lesson 12: Visiting an Emergency Room:
Pronunciation Exercise
(pair activity)

Copy the following lists of words for Partner B. Partner A's is on pages 104-105. Where it says "Listen and check" put a check mark by the word your partner pronounces. Where it says "Pronounce" say the word that is underlined, and your partner will put a check mark by that word. *Do not look at your partner's page.* When you are finished, correct your answers. If you don't know how to pronounce a word, ask the teacher.

PARTNER B

1. Pronounce:

    <u>blood</u>

    brood

    bud

2. Listen and check:

    forum   _____

    from   _____

    form   _____

3. Pronounce:

    shake

    <u>shock</u>

    shook

4. Listen and check:

    hard   _____

    heart   _____

    heard   _____

5. Pronounce:

    scared

    scored

    <u>scarred</u>

6. Listen and check:

    chafing   _____

    choking   _____

    shaking   _____

7. Pronounce:

    <u>drowning</u>

    droning

    draining

8. Listen and check:

    fear   _____

    far   _____

    fair   _____

9. Pronounce:

    pain

    pan

    <u>pine</u>

10. Listen and check:

    passions   _____

    patients   _____

    patents   _____

11. Pronounce:

<u>fission</u>

fashion

vision

12. Listen and check:

stale _____

style _____

steal _____

13. Pronounce:

<u>lose</u>

loose

rose

14. Listen and check:

rum _____

room _____

loom _____

Emergency!
(pair activity)

Ask your partner for the information for your blank boxes. Use the conversation below. Write the information in your boxes. *Do not look at your partner's page*

PARTNER B

A: What has _____ done?

B: He/she has _____.

A: Where did he/she _____?

B: He/she _____ in _____

Name	What he/she did	Where
Jack Tripper		in the lobby
Mary Wanna	took a drug overdose	
Dee Livery		in the parking lot
Kent Cutwright	cut his arm badly	

Lesson 15: Childhood Diseases: *Contagious Diseases*

(pair activity)

Ask your partner for the information for your blank boxes. Use the conversation below. Write the information in your boxes. *Do not look at your partner's page*

PARTNER B

A: What is/are _____'s _____?

B: His/Her _____ is/are _____.

Name	Symptoms	Disease	Treatment
Ivan		mumps	
Susanna	high fever, sore throat, swelling in neck		antibiotic, non-spirin drug
Irene	fever, itchy red spots on skin		
David		measles	rest in a dark room, drink fluids, non-aspirin drug

Lesson 16: Lice: *Pronunciation Exercise*
(pair activity)

Copy the following lists of words for Partner B. Partner A's are on page 140. Where it says "Listen and check" put a check mark by the word your partner pronounces. Where it says "Pronounce" say the word that is underlined, and your partner will put a check mark by that word. *Do not look at your partner's page.* When you are finished, correct your answers. If you don't know how to pronounce a word, ask the teacher.

PARTNER B

1. Pronounce:

   higher

   here

   hair

2. Listen and check:

   lies _____

   lice _____

   rice _____

3. Pronounce:

   ditty

   dirty

   thirty

4. Listen and check:

   nurse _____

   nerds _____

   Norse _____

5. Pronounce:

   scalp

   escape

   scald

6. Listen and check:

   vacation _____

   vaccination _____

   back in the
   station _____

7. Pronounce:

   height

   high

   hate

8. Listen and check:

   vice _____

   bites _____

   buys _____

9. Pronounce

   lash

   rush

   rash

10. Listen and check:

    blush _____

    brush _____

    bush _____

11. Pronounce:

sprit

spread

<u>sprayed</u>

12. Listen and check:

scrapes _____

scraps _____

scratch _____

13. Pronounce:

flea

flew

<u>fly</u>

14. Listen and check:

heed _____

head _____

hid _____

Lesson 20: AIDS:
Pronunciation Exercise: Past Tense with –ed
(pair activity)

There are three ways to pronounce the "–ed" at the end of past tense verbs, One is like the sound "t" (example: "wished"), one is like "id" (example: "started"), and the third is simply the sound of "d" (example: borrowed). Copy the following chart and then ask your partner how to pronounce the past tense verb forms. Repeat the correct pronunciation and write the verb in the correct column on the verb chart. You have half the information; your partner has the other half. So that you really listen and learn the correct pronunciation, be sure not to look at your partner's chart until after you are finished.

Partner B's question: How do you pronounce the past tense of _____?

	Present	Past		
		–id	–t	–d
Ask	1. care			
Listen and pronounce	2. like		liked	
Ask	3. tend			
Listen and pronounce	4. repeat	repeated		
Ask	5. finish			
Listen and pronounce	6. play			played
Ask	7. miss			

	Present	Past		
		–id	–t	–d
Listen and pronounce	8. decide	decided		
Ask	9. call			
Listen and pronounce	10. ask		asked	
Ask	11. want			
Listen and pronounce	12. share			shared
Ask	13. notice			
Listen and pronounce	14. yell			yelled
Ask	15. learn			
Listen and pronounce	16. wait	waited		
Ask	17. touch			

Lesson 21: Annual Examination: *Formulating Questions*
(pair activity)

This exercise is designed to help you put words in the correct order for questions. When your partner asks you a question, do not answer it until the question is phrased correctly. You will have the correct phrasing on your page when you are the listener. Listen carefully. You may help your partner phrase it correctly, but do not answer the question until your partner says the question correctly.

PARTNER B

1. Listen and answer (when the question is phrased correctly):
   "Do you have any children?"
2. Ask your partner if he/she has any present illnesses.
   Your partner's answer: _____
3. Listen and answer (when the question is phrased correctly):
   "Have you ever smoked?"
4. Ask your partner when his/her last physical examination was.
   Your partner's answer: _____
5. Listen and answer (when the question is phrased correctly):

"Have you been in the hospital in the last five years?"

6. Ask your partner when he/she thinks they will find a cure for AIDS.
Your partner's answer: _____

7. Listen and answer (when the question is phrased correctly):
"How did you get to this class?"

8. Ask your partner why he/she took this class.
Your partner's answer: _____

9. Listen and answer (when the question is phrased correctly):
"Why don't you like to go to the doctor?"

10. Ask your partner if he/she would like to lend you fifty dollars.
Your partner's answer: _____

Lesson 22: Breast Examination: *Reflexive Pronouns*
(pair activity)

Study the following list of reflexive pronouns:

Singular	Plural
myself	ourselves
yourself	yourselves
himself	themselves
herself	
itself	

PARTNER B

Refer to the list on page 231 and fill in this chart. *Do not look at your partner's chart.*

Ask your partner, "What did _____ do?"

Person	Activity	Reflexive Pronoun	Rest of Sentence

PARTNER B

Ask your partner, "What did _____ do?"

Person	Activity	Reflexive Pronoun	Rest of Sentence
Theresa	gave	_____	a day off.
Tomas	_____	himself	shaving.
We	_____	ourselves	on our good grades.
They	watched	_____	on television.
The dog	_____	itself	behind its ear.
You	considered	_____	one of the family.
You two	_____	yourselves	on the ice.
I	sent	_____	a present.
Ana and Ed	_____	themselves	in the wall mirror.
He	prepared	_____	for the struggle ahead.

Pronunciation Exercise

(pair activity)

Copy the following lists of words for Partner B. Partner A's is on pages 208-209.). Where it says "Listen and check" put a check mark by the word your partner pronounces. Where it says "Pronounce" say the word that is underlined, and your partner will put a check mark by that word. *Do not look at your partner's page.* When you are finished, correct your answers. If you don't know how to pronounce a word, ask the teacher.

PARTNER B

1. Pronounce:

<u>disk</u>

risk

list

2. Listen and check:

sheared   _____

share   _____

shared   _____

3. Pronounce:

fright

<u>flight</u>

fight

4. Listen and check:

quite   _____

cute   _____

quit   _____

5. Pronounce:

<u>raw</u>

low

law

6. Listen and check:

blend   _____

plan   _____

bland   _____

7. Pronounce:

bane

been

<u>bean</u>

8. Listen and check:

police   _____

bodice   _____

policy   _____

9. Pronounce:

plowed

prude

<u>proud</u>

10. Listen and check:

expensive   _____

expansive   _____

especially   _____

11. Listen and check:

sign   _____

seen   _____

sighed   _____

12. Pronounce:

very

<u>berry</u>

belly

13. Listen and check:

ides   _____

AIDS   _____

eyes   _____

14. Pronounce:

visa

<u>busy</u>

visit